Assessing Essential Skills of Veterinary Technology Students

Assessing Essential Skills of Veterinary Technology Students

Fourth Edition

Edited by

Lisa E. Schenkel, DVM, CCRT, CVMA
Mercy University, 555 Broadway Dobbs Ferry, NY 10522

Amanda Colón, DVM
Mercy University, 555 Broadway Dobbs Ferry, NY 10522

Sandra Lynn Bertholf, MS, LVT
Mercy University, 555 Broadway Dobbs Ferry, NY 10522

Sabrina Timperman, DVM
Mercy University, 555 Broadway Dobbs Ferry, NY 10522

Laurie J. Buell, MS, LVT
Scottsdale, Arizona

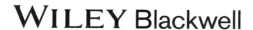

Library of Congress Cataloging-in-Publication Data is applied for:

Cover Design: Wiley
Cover Images: Courtesy of Kenneth Gabrielsen, Courtesy of Sandra Bertholf, Courtesy of Lisa E. Schenkel, Courtesy of Amanda Colón, Courtesy of Sabrina Timperman

Set in 9.5/12.5pt STIXTwoText by Straive, Pondicherry, India

SKY10081011_080124

To all of our veterinary patients, past, present, and future, and to those who choose to rise to the challenge to give them a voice.

Contents

List of Contributors

Laurie J. Buell, MS, LVT
Veterinary Technologist
Former Associate Professor and Program Director
Veterinary Technology Program
Mercy University
Dobbs Ferry, NY

Sandra Lynn Bertholf, MS, LVT
Associate Program Director
Assistant Professor
Veterinary Technology Program
Mercy University
Dobbs Ferry, NY

Veterinary Technologist
Animal Medical of New City
New City, NY

Amanda Colón, DVM
Assistant Professor
Veterinary Technology Program
Mercy University
Dobbs Ferry, NY

Associate Veterinarian
Thornwood Animal Hospital
Thornwood, NY

Howard Gittelman, MS, DVM
Hospital Director
Animal Medical of New City
New City, NY

Annmarie Gonzalez, BS, LVT
Veterinary Technologist
Red Bank Veterinary Hospital
Tinton Falls, NJ

Adjunct Instructor
Veterinary Technology Program
Mercy University
Dobbs Ferry, NY

Jacquelyn Hickey, BS, LVT
Veterinary Technologist
Animal Medical of New City
New City, NY

Adjunct Instructor
Veterinary Technology Program
Mercy University
Dobbs Ferry, NY

Lisa E. Schenkel, DVM, CCRT, CVMA
Program Director
Assistant Professor
Veterinary Technology Program
Mercy University
Dobbs Ferry, NY

Associate Veterinarian
Animal Medical of New City
New City, NY

Nina Slivinsky, LVT, LATg
Facility Manager
Department of Comparative Medicine
New York Medical College
Valhalla, New York

Sabrina Timperman, DVM
Associate Professor
Veterinary Technology Program
Mercy University
Dobbs Ferry, NY

Preface

The importance of a qualified, skilled, and critically thinking veterinary technician/technologist on the veterinary team cannot be overstated. In today's modern society where medicine is becoming more advanced and complex, a team of health care providers who work collaboratively, each contributing their expertise to provide the best possible care for their patients, is the ideal in any veterinary facility. As part of the journey of becoming a veterinary technician/technologist, the development of solid technical skills, critical thinking, and problem solving is essential. Everyone agrees how important it is to know how to complete a task, but that knowledge alone is not enough. Understanding how to work through a problem, analyze important data, come to appropriate conclusions, and determine the most appropriate response are skills all veterinary professionals must strive to attain. As veterinary technology educators, the goal is to guide our students, teaching them the required veterinary knowledge while at the same time providing the education that supports the development of their ability to think through problems, reason out correct interpretations, and determine the most beneficial course of action. As educators, the job of teaching these skills is crucial, but of equal importance is the role of assessing skills acquisition in a manner that is commiserate with current standards of care. Veterinary technology programs across the nation strive to meet both these objectives. The current landscape of veterinary technology education has changed over the years. Currently, there are 222 veterinary technology programs accredited by the American Veterinary Medical Association Committee on Veterinary Technician Education and Activities (AVMA CVTEA®). Of these, 28 are four-year programs, 10 are online programs, and the remaining are two-year programs. Regardless of what type of program a student attends, the goals and objectives are the same. All programs strive to teach their students the skills they will need to be successful members of the veterinary team. While differences in programs are inevitable, the goal is steadfast: Prepare each student to be the best technician/technologist possible so they can provide exemplary care.

Attaining this goal is of the utmost importance for veterinary technology educators, their students, and the profession. Variability exists in how different programs tackle the challenges of educating veterinary technology students, as it should. Each program is unique and needs to navigate how best to teach their population of students. What is consistent across programs is the decision-making skills and tasks that each veterinary technology student must attain to graduate from an AVMA CVTEA accredited program. The evaluation of any student's competency in completing these skills successfully, however, can inherently be subjective. It is important, therefore, to create a way to objectively evaluate students, ensuring that any student who graduates from an AVMA CVTEA accredited program has attained the level of competency consistent with an entry-level veterinary technician/technologist. This book was created with this goal in mind. It provides educators with explicit, up-to-date assessment criteria for both the hands-on-skills and the decision-making capabilities considered essential as of August 2023 (Committee on Veterinary Technician Education and Activities, 2023).

Employers need to know the level of competency that graduates from any AVMA CVTEA accredited program have in technical and cognitive skills to make employment decisions. Ensuring that all students who graduate from AVMA CVTEA accredited programs have been assessed with criteria that meets current standards of care will help elevate the profession and highlight why it is imperative to have an educated veterinary technician/technologist on every veterinary team.

To develop the assessment criteria in this book, the contributors used their experience teaching in a four-year, bachelor-of-science-degree program, along with their many years of practice in the veterinary field. The contributors hope this text will be a useful resource for all veterinary technology educators and students. Anticipated uses for this text include:

- A guide for students, describing the criteria that will be used to assess the acquisition of the hands-on-skills and decision-making capabilities needed for them to graduate from an AVMA CVTEA accredited program.
- A resource for veterinary technology educators to ensure objective assessment of the hands-on and decision-making capabilities required by the AVMA CVTEA ensuring entry-level competency for all graduates of AVMA CVTEA accredited programs.
- A model for standard competency that veterinary technology programs can use to ensure graduates are achieving entry level competency of the AVMA CVTEA required skills.

Lisa E. Schenkel
Sandra Lynn Bertholf
Amanda Colón
Sabrina Timperman
December 2023

References

Committee on Veterinary Technician Education and Activities. (2023, August). *CVTEA Accreditation Policies and Procedures – Appendix G*. Retrieved from American Veterinary Medical Association: https://www.avma.org/education/center-for-veterinary-accreditation/committee-veterinary-technician-education-activities/cvtea-accreditation-policies-and-procedures-appendix-g

Committee on Veterinary Technician Education and Activities. (2023). *Programs accredited by the AVMA Committee on Veterinary Technician Education and Activities (CVTEA)*. Retrieved from American Veterinary Medical Association: https://www.avma.org/Professional Development/Education/Accreditation/Programs/Pages/vettech-programs.aspx

About the Companion Website

This book is accompanied by a companion website:

www.wiley.com/go/Schenkel/AssessingEssentialSkillsofVeterinaryTechnologyStudents4e

There, you will find valuable material designed to enhance your learning:

- Excel

- The student displays knowledge of how to recognize severe or abnormal grieving and shows familiarity with appropriate resources for professional assistance.

23) **The student demonstrates understanding of how to effectively communicate relevant and accurate information to clients and team members.**
    - Based on the patient, client, staff, and the situation at hand, the student displays understanding of how to effectively communicate in order to gather and relay relevant and accurate information in a timely and appropriate manner.

1.3 Ethics and Jurisprudence

24) **The student demonstrates clear understanding of laws pertaining to each member of the veterinary health care team and recognizes the necessity to observe them.**
    - The student demonstrates knowledge and practical understanding of the applicable state practice act for veterinary technicians/technologists and assistants, in states where one exists.
    - The student displays knowledge of the applicable state practice act for veterinarians.
    - The student demonstrates knowledge and practical understanding of the code of ethics for veterinary technicians/technologists, as developed by the ethics committee of the National Association of Veterinary Technicians in America (NAVTA) (National Association of Veterinary Technicians in America, 2023).
    - The student demonstrates appreciation of the potential legal and professional ramifications of violating federal and state laws that pertain to each member of the veterinary health care team.

25) **In all interactions with clients and staff members, the student demonstrates knowledge of how to behave professionally and ethically in light of legal boundaries.**
    - The student demonstrates appreciation of the potential legal ramifications of client and staff interactions.
    - The student demonstrates understanding of what is and is not appropriate and professional to discuss with clients.

26) **The student exhibits dedication to providing high-quality patient care.**
    - The student demonstrates the requisite knowledge as well as motivation needed to provide high-caliber patient care.
    - The student demonstrates appreciation of the importance of continuing education in providing high-quality care.
    - The student displays recognition of the ethical responsibility to provide high-quality patient care.

27) **The student displays understanding of how to maintain confidentiality as it pertains to client and patient information.**
    - The student demonstrates a clear understanding of the meaning of confidentiality as it pertains to clients and patients, recognizing its essential nature and respecting it at all times.
    - The student shows understanding of legal and ethical considerations regarding confidentiality.
    - As stated in the NAVTA Code of Ethics, the student protects "confidential information provided by clients" (National Association of Veterinary Technicians in America, 2023).

28) **The student demonstrates the ability to make informed decisions in accordance with ethical and legal boundaries.**
    - The student demonstrates the ability to make appropriate decisions with regards to client interactions and patient care that are in compliance with the ethical and legal standards of current veterinary practice.

References

American Veterinary Medical Association. (n/d). *The Veterinarian-Client-Patient Relationship* (VCPR). Retrieved July 23, 2023, from AVMA. org: https://www.avma.org/resources-tools/pet-owners/petcare/veterinarian-client-patient-relationship-vcpr

Bertholf, S. (2017). Veterinary management. In *Assessing Essential Skills of Veterinary Technology Students*, 3rd e. (ed. L. J. Buell, L. E. Schenkel, and S. Timperman), 1–4. Ames: John Wiley & Sons, Inc.

National Association of Veterinary Technicians in America. (2023). *About NAVTA-National Association of Veterinary Technicians in America*. Retrieved July 23, 2023, from NAVTA.net: https://navta.net/policies/#:~:text=Code%20of%20Ethics,-Veterinary%20technicians%20shall&text=Veterinary%20technicians%20shall%20prevent%20and,the%20public%20about%20these%20diseases.

2

Pharmacology
Lisa E. Schenkel, DVM, CCRT, CVMA

2.1 Pharmacologic Fundamentals of Drug Administration

1) **The student displays knowledge of how to correctly comply with the veterinarian's pharmacy (medication) orders, both written and verbal.**
   - The student displays understanding of the meaning of the terms *dose, dosage strength, dosage interval,* and *dosage* (or *dosage regimen*) and how to implement them correctly in the clinical setting.
   - The student shows knowledge of terms used in medication orders, including appropriate abbreviations, and how to apply them correctly in the clinical setting.
   - The student recognizes the importance of verifying patient identification, selecting the correct drug in the proper dosage form, and administering the prescribed dose via the appropriate route at the correct time.
2) **The student demonstrates knowledge of various drug categories, mechanisms of action, major therapeutic uses, and common, clinically significant adverse effects.**
   - The student demonstrates basic understanding of the clinical pathology underlying disease processes treated by frequently used drugs.
   - The student demonstrates fundamental understanding of primary mechanisms of action of commonly used drugs. Based on this knowledge, the student displays the basic ability to reason out the drug's major therapeutic effects and applications, contraindications, and clinically important, mechanism-based adverse effects.
   - The student identifies clinically relevant, idiosyncratic adverse effects of commonly used drugs.
3) **The student describes proper techniques for preparing and administering vaccines, as well as explains common adverse effects associated with vaccine administration.**
   - The student displays understanding of the basic immunologic concepts underlying immunization.
   - The student recognizes the importance of:
     1) Using a new, sterile syringe and needle for each patient.
     2) Only using diluents provided or recommended by the manufacturer.
     3) Not mixing vaccines in the same syringe, unless recommended by the manufacturer.

Assessing Essential Skills of Veterinary Technology Students, Fourth Edition. Edited by Lisa E. Schenkel, Amanda Colón, Sandra Lynn Bertholf, Sabrina Timperman, and Laurie J. Buell.
© 2024 John Wiley & Sons, Inc. Published 2024 by John Wiley & Sons, Inc.
Companion website: www.wiley.com/go/Schenkel/AssessingEssentialSkillsofVeterinaryTechnologyStudents4e

4) Using recommended sites and routes of administration for individual vaccines and noting vaccination sites in patient records.

5) Administering vaccines within an appropriate time frame after reconstitution.

6) Administering the entire recommended dose to the patient.

- The student demonstrates the ability to identify and explain potential adverse reactions to vaccines, including, but not limited to, transient lethargy, low-grade fever, vomiting, diarrhea, anaphylaxis, local inflammation at the injection site, granulomas, and vaccination-site sarcomas.

- The student demonstrates the ability to distinguish clinically significant adverse reactions to vaccination and recognizes the urgent need for an appropriate response, including the immediate notification of a supervisor.

4) **The student accurately calculates drug doses and dosages, correctly using weights and measures.**

- The student demonstrates understanding of relevant systems of weights and measures, including metric, apothecary and household systems, and describes their appropriate uses in the clinical setting.

- The student accurately performs unit conversions, including, but not limited to:

1) Conversions between systems of measurement, such as pounds to kilograms.

2) Conversions within systems of measurement, as in milliliters to liters.

- The student correctly calculates drug doses.

- The student accurately identifies and correctly uses the supplied dosage strength (e.g., mg/mL, mg/tab) to convert from units of dose (e.g., mg, mEq) to units for administration (e.g., tablets, mL).

- The student correctly measures doses, accurately reading calibrations on syringe barrels and droppers.

5) **The student demonstrates knowledge of appropriate routes and methods of administration for commonly used drugs. If more than one administration route and/or method is commonly used for a drug, the student displays knowledge of the correct clinical indications for each.**

- The student demonstrates understanding of comparative rates of absorption and onsets of effect of various administration routes.

- The student shows knowledge of drug types that should not be given subcutaneously or intramuscularly (e.g., agents that are extremely acidic or alkaline, vesicants, etc.).

- The student displays knowledge of drugs that should not be administered intravenously (e.g., any drug not labeled for IV administration, repository preparations, suspensions or solutions with any sign of precipitation, etc.).

- In selecting an appropriate route and method of drug administration, the student demonstrates the ability to consider the individual patient, the veterinarian's instructions, and the prescribed drug to achieve the greatest therapeutic response while minimizing potential adverse responses. For example, the student considers individual patient status, correctly explaining that oral administration generally is contraindicated in a vomiting or dyspneic animal.

- The student explains the proper administration of drugs by prescribed routes, including common enteral and parenteral routes, at prescribed dosage intervals, describing safe and effective techniques.

  - The student correctly describes commonly used enteral and parenteral administration routes.

  - The student describes proper techniques for administering oral medications. The student demonstrates understanding of how to avoid complications such as esophageal stricture by administering an appropriate volume of water by mouth, following administration of oral tablets and capsules.

– The student explains correct techniques for administering drugs parenterally. The student identifies appropriate muscles and landmarks for IM drug administration. The student identifies appropriate veins for IV drug administration. The student identifies appropriate sites for SC drug administration.

6) **The student displays knowledge of how to carefully monitor patients for therapeutic responses and adverse reactions to drugs.**

- The student properly defines the terms *therapeutic response, adverse reaction,* and *side effect.*
- The student demonstrates the basic ability to recognize therapeutic effects of drugs and to distinguish them from adverse effects of drugs.

7) **The student demonstrates the ability to accurately enter all information pertaining to drug and/or vaccine administration in patients' medical records.**

- The student displays the ability to precisely record information in the patient's record, including, but not limited to, the name of the drug, the dose administered, the route of administration, the site of administration, and when and by whom the medication or vaccine was administered.
- The student uses correct drug names and properly uses veterinary abbreviations, where appropriate.

8) **The student displays knowledge of DEA regulations regarding scheduled (controlled) substances.**

- The student correctly defines the terms *controlled or scheduled drug.* The student demonstrates practical understanding of the classification of controlled drugs into five schedules. The student accurately identifies common controlled drugs used therapeutically in practice and correctly classifies them as to Schedule (II–V) (Drug Enforcement Administration, 2023).
- The student demonstrates knowledge and appreciates the importance of compliance with all federal and state regulations governing the purchase, storage, administration, dispensing, labeling, inventorying, and disposing of scheduled drugs.
- The student describes the proper disposal of unused or expired controlled substances, in accordance with state and federal regulations.
- The student completes a controlled substance inventory log, accurately recording each use in the controlled substance inventory log and in the patient's medical record. (The student records both the amount drawn up and the amount administered when these quantities differ.)

9) **The student demonstrates knowledge of all state and federal regulations applicable to the purchase, storage, handling, dispensing, administration, disposal, and inventorying of drugs, biologics, pesticides, insecticides, and hazardous wastes derived from these substances.**

- The student displays proficiency in accurately identifying and differentiating drugs, biologics, pesticides, insecticides, and hazardous waste.
- The student demonstrates practical knowledge of state and federal regulations pertaining to these substances. This includes the roles of the Food and Drug Administration (FDA) in overseeing drug evaluation, approval and marketing, the United States Department of Agriculture (USDA) in regulating biologics (including vaccines, antitoxins, etc.), and the Drug Enforcement Administration (DEA) in enforcing federal laws and rules pertaining to controlled drugs.

- The student demonstrates knowledge of potential safety concerns when working with and around pharmaceutical agents, biologics, insecticides, pesticides, and hazardous wastes derived from these agents.
- The student displays appreciation of the importance of precisely following manufacturers' recommendations for the proper handling, storage, administration and disposal of pharmaceutical agents, biologics, insecticides, and pesticides.

10) **The student demonstrates knowledge of how to properly prepare medications for administration.**
- The student accurately reads drug labels, displaying knowledge of proprietary and non-proprietary drug names and dosage strengths. The student shows knowledge of how to select the correct (prescribed) drug and dosage strength.
- The student demonstrates understanding of the importance of carefully checking the label at least three times.
- The student recognizes the need to check all drug containers for cracks, foreign matter, precipitation, color changes, expiration dates, reconstitution dates, and other evidence of expiration or non-viability.
- The student displays appreciation of the need to wash their hands prior to handling injectable agents and maintains aseptic technique, when appropriate.
- The student demonstrates knowledge of how to select or prepare drugs in the prescribed form, correctly reconstituting drugs to desired dosage strengths when appropriate.
- The student selects appropriate equipment for drug administration, including:
  1) Choosing syringe size based on the volume of the dose and/or type (or dosage concentration) of drug. For example, using a 1 cc (tuberculin)

syringe for a volume of 0.25 cc or using a U-100 insulin syringe for U-100 insulin.
  2) Choosing a needle gauge based on the quantity and type of fluid, administration route, and size, species, and age of the animal.

2.2 Pharmacy Essentials of Drug Dispensing

11) **The student displays the ability to properly prepare prescribed drugs to dispense to clients.**
- The student demonstrates knowledge of the names of commonly used agents.
- The student displays knowledge of veterinary terminology and abbreviations used in medication orders and prescriptions.
- The student accurately performs appropriate dosage calculations, correctly using weights and measures.
- The student demonstrates the ability to properly prepare drugs in the prescribed form, dose, dosage strength, and number of doses.

12) **The student demonstrates knowledge of the differences between prescription and over-the-counter drugs and abides by all laws and regulations applicable to each.**
- The student demonstrates understanding of the concept that no drug is free of risks, and that all drugs are associated with potential hazardous or undesirable effects.
- The student displays knowledge that prescription (legend) drugs are considered by the Food and Drug Administration (FDA) to be unsafe for use, except under the supervision of a veterinarian, physician, or other practitioner licensed to prescribe drugs. The student demonstrates knowledge of over-the-counter (OTC) drugs as those that do not require the

supervision of a licensed practitioner to be used and do not require a prescription to be purchased.

- The student shows knowledge of FDA labeling, including, but not limited to, approved indications, contraindications, warnings, precautions, adverse reactions, dosage, and administration.
- The student demonstrates knowledge of the Animal Medicinal Drug Use Clarification Act (AMDUCA), as well as its provisions and requirements for extra-label drug use in animals (Food and Drug Administration, 2023).

13) **The student demonstrates an understanding of how to maintain a controlled drug log in accordance with federal and state regulations.**
   - The student shows understanding that the controlled drug logs must be bound logbooks and not loose leaf.
   - The student demonstrates knowledge that the logs for schedule II drugs must be maintained separately from the logs of schedule III–V drugs. The student also shows awareness that maintaining a separate log for each controlled drug that is dispensed or administered may be more efficient.
   - The student displays awareness that controlled drug logs must be readily retrievable.
   - The student correctly explains how to document controlled drugs that have been administered or dispensed in the controlled drug log, including all of the required information as federally mandated (at a minimum: drug name, container size, strength of medication, bottle number, date of dispensation, explanation of use, lot number (if available), expiration date, amount added to logbook, amount used, running balance, initials of authorized employee, and witness initials for wasting) (Title 21 Code of Federal Regulations, 2023).

- The student describes how to reconcile the running balance in the controlled drug log with the in-hospital controlled drug stock.
- The student displays awareness that controlled drug logs must be kept for a minimum of two years according to federal regulations and that some state regulations may require that logs be kept for a longer period of time.

14) **The student displays the ability to provide clients with appropriate, complete, and accurate information when dispensing drugs.**
   - The student demonstrates adequate knowledge of commonly used therapeutic agents, including their proper handling, storage, administration, and therapeutic indications. The student demonstrates awareness of common adverse drug reactions and drug interactions.
   - The student displays the ability to communicate necessary drug information to clients in a manner that maximizes client understanding, compliance with prescribed therapy, and safety for both the client and the patient.
   - The student labels medications correctly and legibly, with proper directions to the client.
     - The student lists complete, required information on prescription drug labels, including: the name, address, and phone number of the veterinarian; the client's name, address, and phone number; identification of the animal, species, number of animals (if treating a group, herd, or flock); the date of treatment, prescribing or dispensing of the drug; the established name of the drug (active ingredient); the unit strength, dose, dosage frequency and duration; the route of administration; the quantity to be dispensed; the expiration date; precautionary information; and the number

of refills, if any (American Veterinary Medical Association, 2023).

- For food-producing animals, the student shows awareness that slaughter-withdrawal and/or milk-withholding times must be included, if applicable.
- The student demonstrates understanding that state law and other regulations may require more or other information than previously listed before.
- The student displays knowledge of labelling information required for extra-label use of drugs (Food and Drug Administration, 2023).

References

American Veterinary Medical Association. (2023). *Use of Prescription Drugs in Veterinary Medicine*. Retrieved September 19, 2023, from American Veterinary Medical Association: www.avma.org/resources-tools/avma-policies/use-prescription-drugs-veterinary-medicine

Buell, L. J. and Schenkel, L. E. (2017). Pharmacology. In *Assessing Essential Skills of Veterinary Technology Students*, 3rd e. (ed. L. J. Buell, L. E. Schenkel, and S. Timperman), 5–8. Ames: John Wiley & Sons, Inc.

Drug Enforcement Administration (2023). *Drug Scheduling*. Retrieved September 18, 2023, from United States Drug Enforcement Administration: www.dea.gov/drug-information/drug-scheduling.

Food and Drug Administration. (2023, August 31). *Extralabel Drug Use in Animals*. Retrieved September 18, 2023, from National Archives and Records Administration: www.ecfr.gov/current/title-21/chapter-I/subchapter-E/part-530.

Title 21 Code of Federal Regulations. (2023, August 31). *Maintenance of Records and Inventories*. Retrieved September 18, 2023, from National Archives and Records Administration: https://www.ecfr.gov/current/title-21/chapter-II/part-1304/subject-group-ECFR64b4002fc681198/section-1304.04.

3

Medical Nursing

Lisa E. Schenkel, DVM, CCRT, CVMA, Sandra Lynn Bertholf, MS, LVT, and Howard Gittelman, MS, DVM

3.1 Assessment of the Veterinary Patient

1) **The student displays the ability to effectively acquire subjective and objective information that permits accurate assessment of the patient's status.**
   - The student's actions show that they consider safety of personnel and patients to be of paramount importance in patient assessment.
   - The student is careful to thoroughly wash their hands between handling animals, before donning sterile gloves, and after contact with body fluids or tissues.
   - The student displays an understanding of how to obtain a thorough, relevant patient history and record it in the animal's medical record.
   - The student successfully obtains accurate, objective patient data and makes correct notations in the animal's medical record.

2) **The student displays knowledge of common domestic animal species and breeds.**
   - The student shows the ability to recognize the species of common domestic animals and differentiate various breeds.

- The student displays the ability to identify the sex of common domestic species. The student describes behavioral and anatomic characteristics of the various breeds of common domestic animals.

3) **The student demonstrates the ability to explain and use common methods of animal identification.**
   - The student displays appreciation of the importance of properly identifying the patient upon admission to the facility and prior to every treatment and/or procedure.
   - The student shows knowledge that patient identification includes confirmation of the patient's name, age, sex, reproductive status, vaccine status, medical history (including reason for hospitalization), and pertinent behavioral information –for example, "will bite" or level of arousal according to the Fear Aggression Scale (Martin, D and Martin K, 2022).
   - The student displays knowledge of how to properly label and use all appropriate facility equipment, such as neck bands and cage cards, to identify patients.
   - The student demonstrates knowledge of microchips, including implantation techniques, use of handheld scanners, and

Assessing Essential Skills of Veterinary Technology Students, Fourth Edition. Edited by Lisa E. Schenkel, Amanda Colón, Sandra Lynn Bertholf, Sabrina Timperman, and Laurie J. Buell.
© 2024 John Wiley & Sons, Inc. Published 2024 by John Wiley & Sons, Inc.
Companion website: www.wiley.com/go/Schenkel/AssessingEssentialSkillsofVeterinaryTechnologyStudents4e

the availability of different types of microchips.

- The student shows awareness of the use of tattoos as identification and common sites utilized.
- The student displays knowledge of identification of the reproductive status of animals such as clipping the left ear of cats and tattooing the ventral abdomen of dogs, as well as knowledge of when such identification methods are appropriately employed.
- The student demonstrates knowledge of identification techniques for large animals, such as ear tagging, branding, and electronic identification.
- The student displays the ability to explain the advantages and disadvantages of common identification procedures.

4) **The student displays knowledge of normal behaviors of various species and demonstrates understanding of how to recognize and assess the body language and behaviors of various species, including through the use of pain assessment scales.**
- The student can describe what constitutes normal behaviors of various species.
- The student displays an understanding of how the environment or situation (such as being examined or hospitalized) can affect the behaviors of various species, as well as individual patients.
- The student demonstrates knowledge of the body language of various species as it relates to normal versus abnormal behaviors and the status of the veterinary patient.
- The student displays an awareness of how to relate body language of various species to the level of fear, anxiety, and stress of the veterinary patient (Martin, D and Martin K, 2022).
- The student shows the ability to describe behaviors that may indicate the presence of pain in various species.
- The student displays an awareness of the different types of pain scales used for various species and the importance of the

consistent use of pain scales in veterinary patient assessment.
- The student demonstrates an understanding of how to use pain scales in the assessment of veterinary patients.

5) **The student humanely utilizes appropriate stress-reducing techniques when restraining cats, dogs, and various other species for procedures.**
- The student accurately assesses the patient's body language and temperament.
- The student utilizes appropriate restraint techniques when needed, based on species, size, temperament, level of arousal, medical status, and procedure to be performed.
- The student restrains various species in a manner that promotes calmness and avoids stress and injury, while properly controlling the movement of the patient.
- The student demonstrates awareness of the organization that promotes Fear Free® techniques for veterinary professionals (https://fearfreepets.com/).

6) **The student effectively, safely, and properly encages and removes dogs and cats from cages.**
- The student approaches the cage carefully, accurately assesses the animal's temperament based on its body language and behavior, and safely removes and encages the animal.
- The student avoids stressing the animal, applying only appropriate restraint techniques as needed.

7) **The student effectively, safely, and correctly affixes muzzles on dogs.**
- The student displays familiarity with different muzzle types, including basket muzzles, brachycephalic-specific muzzles, and rope or gauze.
- The student appropriately restrains and safely applies the appropriate muzzles to dogs.

8) **The student effectively, safely, and correctly affixes Elizabethan collars.**
- The student describes various styles of Elizabethan collars (E-collars) and the advantages and disadvantages of each type.

- The student selects an E-collar of an appropriate size based on the animal's size, condition, and procedure.
- The student correctly assembles the E-collar, if required.
- The student effectively restrains the animal and securely affixes the E-collar on the animal, so that it is not too loose or too tight.

9) **The student participates in and can explain how to effectively and correctly employ a restraint pole and other restraint aids.**
   - The student describes various restraint aids and the advantages and disadvantages of each type.
   - The student demonstrates knowledge of how to correctly use a restraint pole.
   - The student displays knowledge of how to correctly and appropriately use other restraint aides, such as towels and gloves.
   - The student participates in the application of the appropriate restraint aid for the patient.

10) **The student effectively, safely, and securely halters, ties, and leads an equine (horses, ponies, mules or donkeys).**
    - The student demonstrates awareness of equine behavior relevant to handling and restraint.
    - The student properly approaches the equine based on correct assessment of the animal's temperament and body language.
    - Using appropriate restraint technique, the student properly applies a halter, tie, and lead rope.
    - The student demonstrates proper use of the lead rope to safely guide the equine.
    - The student displays understanding of when and how to properly use tying as a restraint technique for an equine.

11) **The student participates in effectively, safely, and correctly implementing a mechanical twitch for equine restraint.**
    - The student demonstrates knowledge of proper placement of the twitch on the upper lip, avoiding the delicate inner surface.

- The student displays knowledge of the correct manner of applying and twisting the twitch.
- The student shows understanding of the importance of periodically loosening, tightening, and replacing the twitch.
- The student participates in safely and correctly applying a mechanical twitch for equine restraint.

12) **The student effectively, safely, and correctly implements bovine tail restraint.**
    - The student properly approaches the cow while it is positioned in a stanchion.
    - The student slowly lifts the tail using proper technique.
    - The student applies the appropriate amount of pressure to distract the cow's attention and lowers the tail slowly when the procedure is finished.

13) **The student effectively, safely, and correctly affixes halters to cattle and small ruminants.**
    - The student properly approaches the ruminant from the side when the animal is free-standing, in a chute or in a stanchion.
    - The student applies the halter in a manner that minimizes the chance of injury. The student displays the ability to prevent the small ruminant from slipping out of the halter by holding the animal's nose up while applying the halter.

14) **The student participates in the safe and effective use of a cattle chute.**
    - The student displays knowledge of different chute configurations and their appropriate applications.
    - The student demonstrates knowledge of how to safely direct cattle into a chute.
    - The student displays an understanding of the importance of cleaning in between each period of use and maintaining the chute in good repair to reduce the stress of the cattle.
    - The student participates in the safe and appropriate use of a cattle chute.

15) **The student demonstrates the ability to acquire an accurate and thorough patient history.**
    - The student displays understanding of how to obtain all required information, including, but not limited to, the presenting concern, past medical history, current medications (including dose and frequency of administration), vaccine status, use of preventatives, recent boarding, grooming or travel, reproductive status, and exposure to other animals.
    - The student shows understanding of how to phrase questions appropriately and avoid leading questions.
    - The student displays the ability to legibly and accurately record the history in a systematic, logical sequence, including all available dates.

16) **The student displays competence in safely and accurately determining and recording the temperature of the dog, cat, equine (horse, pony, donkey, or mule), and cow.**
    - The student shows knowledge of different thermometer types and their appropriate uses.
    - The student ensures the patient is appropriately restrained.
    - The student utilizes correct gentle technique, accurately reads the temperature, and records it in the patient's medical record.
    - The student cleans the patient and the thermometer appropriately.

17) **The student displays competence in safely and accurately determining and recording the pulse of the dog, cat, equine (horse, pony, donkey, or mule), cow, and small ruminant.**
    - The student recognizes multiple sites for obtaining the pulse and utilizes the appropriate site based on species and patient.
    - The student palpates the pulse effectively and is able to recognize abnormalities.
    - The student counts the pulse accurately and records the pulse in the patient's medical record.

18) **The student displays competence in safely and accurately determining and recording the respiratory rate of the dog, cat, equine (horse, pony, donkey, or mule), cow, and small ruminant.**
    - The student ensures that the patient is in a relaxed and comfortable position.
    - The student accurately counts the respiratory rate and discerns respiratory effort.
    - The student accurately records the respiratory rate and effort in the patient's medical record.

19) **The student displays competence in safely and accurately ausculting heart and lung sounds in the dog, cat, equine (horse, pony, donkey, or mule), cow, and small ruminant.**
    - The student ensures that the animal is appropriately restrained.
    - The student uses proper auscultation techniques based on species and the conformation of the thorax.
    - The student properly auscults multiple appropriate areas on both sides of the thorax to evaluate heart sounds. The student includes the proper auscultation of the sternum in cats and dogs with a barrel-shaped thorax.
    - The student auscults multiple appropriate areas on both sides of the thorax to evaluate lung sounds.
    - The student recognizes the need to palpate pulses while ausculting the heart and demonstrates the ability to do so correctly.
    - The student correctly differentiates between normal and abnormal heart sounds and rhythms.
    - The student correctly determines the anatomic location of abnormal heart sounds.
    - The student correctly distinguishes between normal and abnormal respiratory sounds, patterns, and effort.

3.2 Nursing Care of the Veterinary Patient

3.2.1 Husbandry of Common Domestic Species

Lisa E. Schenkel, DVM, CCRT, CVMA and Sandra Lynn Bertholf, MS, LVT

31) **The student displays knowledge of how to properly therapeutically bathe, groom, and dip small animals.**
   - The student shows knowledge of various types of therapeutic shampoos and dips, including indications for use.
   - The student demonstrates understanding of how to properly restrain to safely bathe, groom, and dip small animals.
   - The student explains how to properly bathe and apply chemical dips to small animals.
   - The student demonstrates understanding of the importance of protecting the patient's eyes from chemical injury, preventing excess water from entering the external ear canal, and avoiding chemical and thermal injury.
   - The student explains how to properly protect the patient's eyes as well as how to prevent water from entering the external ear canal. The student also describes the appropriate actions to take if the patient's eyes and/or ears are adversely affected.
   - The student displays knowledge of the potential toxic effects of chemical dips and can explain correct dilution techniques.
   - The student shows knowledge of how to correctly utilize protective gear when applying chemical dips and shampoos.
   - The student describes how to appropriately warm and dry animals.
   - The student explains how to properly utilize brushes, combs, and clippers as well as how to remove matted fur without causing damage to the skin.
   - The student explains the importance of checking the ambient temperature and monitoring for signs of hyper- and/or hypothermia, as well as for adverse reactions.

32) **The student correctly trims the claws of dogs and cats.**
   - The student shows knowledge of the fact that dogs and cats have claws (rather than nails).
   - The student displays knowledge of claw anatomy in dogs and cats.
   - The student demonstrates understanding of how to properly restrain dogs and cats to safely trim the claws.
   - The student properly trims the claws of dogs and cats using the correct tools and techniques.
   - The student displays knowledge of the proper use of cauterizing agents/hemostatic techniques, and correctly utilizes them when needed.

33) **The student properly applies equine tail and leg wraps.**
   - The student identifies relevant anatomical structures and anticipates potential problem areas.
   - The student displays understanding of indications for leg and tail wraps.
   - The student properly restrains the patient for wrap application.
   - The student cleans/washes and dries the foot and hoof areas before applying leg wraps.
   - The student properly applies various tail and leg wraps, including gauze, bandage material, and commercially available tail bags.

34) **The student correctly expresses canine anal sacs.**
   - The student accurately identifies the position of anal sacs and ducts.
   - The student demonstrates understanding of potential complications of the procedure, including anal sac rupture and rectal tearing.
   - The student correctly inserts a gloved, lubricated finger into the rectum and completely expresses the anal sacs, using appropriate pressure. The student thoroughly cleans the perianal area.
   - The student correctly distinguishes normal from abnormal anal sac secretions.

35) **The student properly cleans ears and administers otic medications in dogs and cats.**
   - The student demonstrates knowledge of the anatomy of the external ear canal.
   - The student displays understanding of the importance of confirming the presence of an intact tympanic membrane prior to administering any otic cleaning solution or medication.
   - The student demonstrates understanding of the importance of physical or chemical restraint due to the sensitivity of inflamed ears.
   - The student correctly administers ear flushes and/or properly applies appropriate ear cleaning solutions. The student uses appropriate tools and correct techniques for cleaning ears.
   - The student correctly applies appropriate ear medications.
   - The student demonstrates proper technique for medicating ears to the owner and communicates the importance of compliance.

36) **The student effectively carries out sanitation procedures for animal holding and housing areas.**
   - The student displays knowledge of infectious disease transmission, including direct and indirect routes.
   - The student demonstrates understanding of the importance of sanitation and its significance in disease prevention/transmission as well as reducing patient stress.
   - The student shows understanding of the purpose of isolation areas, including the importance of following strict sanitation and disinfection procedures in isolation areas, as well as the importance of preventing animals with no infectious disease from occupying isolation areas.
   - The student uses appropriate personal protective equipment and effectively implements sanitation procedures.
   - The student shows knowledge of the efficacies, relative advantages, and potential disadvantages/toxicities of various disinfectants in use in veterinary facilities.
   - The student appropriately uses various disinfectants.

37) **The student demonstrates knowledge of various methods of permanent identification in common domestic species.**
   - The student demonstrates knowledge of appropriate uses and relative advantages and disadvantages of various methods of identifying large domestic animals, such as tattooing, ear tagging, branding, and electronic methods.
   - The student demonstrates knowledge of permanent identification methods in small animals, such as microchipping and tattooing.

38) **The student demonstrates knowledge of breeding and reproduction procedures.**
   - The student demonstrates knowledge of the estrous cycle in common domestic species and recognizes signs of each stage. In breeding animals, the student shows awareness of how to identify the most appropriate time to breed.
   - The student shows understanding of the care of the female in estrus and is able to explain proper care to the owner.
   - The student demonstrates knowledge of the mating behavior of common domestic species.
   - The student displays awareness of various breeding techniques (such as natural breeding versus artificial insemination) and the advantages and disadvantages of the techniques.
   - The student demonstrates knowledge of the gestation periods of common domestic species. The student explains how to provide appropriate care, including proper nutrition, for the pregnant and lactating female.
   - The student shows knowledge of the signs of approaching parturition. The student demonstrates knowledge of

signs and behaviors associated with stages of labor and birth.

- The student demonstrates knowledge of potential complications associated with labor and birth, clinical signs associated with complications, and how to appropriately intervene if complications develop.
- The student explains how to assist in the normal delivery of newborns.

39) **The student demonstrates understanding of the proper nursing care of neonates and its role in enhancing wellness and reducing risk of disease, injury, and stress.**
- The student demonstrates knowledge of requirements for: maintaining appropriate ambient temperature and hydration; ingestion of colostrum for immune health; proper nutrition and food types; quantity and frequency of feeding; elimination; correct hygiene; proper housing; and socialization.
- The student displays knowledge of common neonatal problems, including dehydration, hypothermia, hypoglycemia, vomiting, diarrhea, elimination difficulties, and anorexia.
- The student shows understanding of proper nursing care for the neonatal problems listed above.
- The student shows the ability to communicate appropriate instructions for neonatal care to owners.

3.2.2 Nutrition of Common Domestic Species

Lisa E. Schenkel, DVM, CCRT, CVMA and Sandra Lynn Bertholf, MS, LVT

40) **For the dog, cat, horse/pony/donkey/ mule, and cow, the student demonstrates knowledge of nutritional requirements for each stage of life.**
- The student demonstrates knowledge of the anatomy and physiology of the gastrointestinal tract and the role it plays in dietary requirements.

- The student shows understanding of appropriate (and inappropriate) dietary components for optimal health in various life stages.
- The student shows the ability to accurately and appropriately calculate resting and daily energy requirements based on the life stage of the animal to maintain a healthy body condition score.
- The student demonstrates the ability to explain nutritional recommendations for various life stages to owners and reinforce owner compliance.

41) **The student demonstrates understanding of the role of nutrients and nutrition in disease states and shows familiarity with therapeutic diets.**
- The student displays understanding of the importance of providing adequate and appropriate nutrition for patients.
- The student shows understanding of enteral and parenteral routes of nutritional support and the appropriate indications for each.
- The student demonstrates knowledge of specific nutritional requirements in common disease states.
- The student displays understanding of the appropriate uses of therapeutic regimens (e.g., prescription diets) in order to enhance recovery and manage chronic diseases.
- The student shows the ability to accurately and appropriately calculate resting and daily energy requirements based on the disease state of the animal.
- The student is able to explain to owners the need for special or therapeutic diets to enhance recovery and manage chronic diseases, and to reinforce owner compliance.

42) **The student demonstrates current knowledge of commonly used nutritional supplements and food additives, including their potential benefits and toxic effects.**

- The student demonstrates awareness of the potential benefits of use of substances classified as nutritional supplements, such as vitamins, minerals, herbs, botanicals, amino acids, and others.
- The student demonstrates understanding of the fact that the FDA does not have authority to require research and FDA approval prior to marketing nutritional supplements. Therefore, manufacturers of nutritional supplements may legally make claims about conditions associated with natural states without FDA approval, even though the efficacy and potential adverse effects have not been identified in controlled studies. In addition, the student shows awareness of the fact that the FDA cannot require removal of nutritional supplements from the market unless the FDA proves significant risk of illness or injury.
- The student demonstrates awareness of the fact that any and all substances, including herbal and/or "all-natural" substances, are potentially associated with toxicities at a certain dose.
- The student shows understanding of the fact that there may be serious interactions between drugs and nutritional supplements and demonstrates knowledge of contraindications of certain nutritional supplements based on patient status.

43) **The student displays knowledge of and is able to identify common poisonous plants.**
- The student identifies common poisonous plants including, but not limited to, *Euphorbia* spp. (poinsettia), *Hydrangea* spp., *Ilex* spp. (holly), *Narcissus* spp. (daffodil), *Nerium* spp. (oleander), *Philodendron* spp., *Phoradendron* spp. (mistletoe), *Toxicodendron* spp. (poison ivy, poison oak), lilies, onions, moldy sweet clover, and so on.
- The student shows knowledge of toxic effects caused by common poisonous plants.

- The student demonstrates familiarity with available resources for poisonous plants and their toxic effects.

44) **The student demonstrates knowledge of and is able to identify common substances that produce toxic effects when ingested.**
- The student displays familiarity with toxicities associated with such substances as commonly used drugs, insecticides (including, but not limited to, organophosphates, limonene, and other citrus oil extracts, etc.), chocolate, caffeine, ethylene glycol, fertilizers, household cleaning products, xylitol, and so on.
- The student describes the pathophysiology, clinical signs, and treatments of common toxic substances in various species.
- The student demonstrates familiarity with available resources for toxic substances, their clinical effects, and treatment.

45) **The student demonstrates understanding of how to develop and effectively communicate hospital nutritional protocols.**
- The student displays knowledge of how to utilize their knowledge of nutritional requirements to create appropriate nutritional protocols for hospitalized patients.
- The student shows understanding of how to effectively communicate nutritional protocols to veterinary staff members in order to ensure continuity of care.
- The student demonstrates understanding of how to appropriately monitor and record daily caloric intake and diet of hospitalized patients.

3.2.3 Therapeutics for Common Domestic Species

Lisa E. Schenkel, DVM, CCRT, CVMA and Sandra Lynn Bertholf, MS, LVT

46) **In light of the veterinarian's directions and the individual patient's characteristics and physical status, the student**

demonstrates understanding of how to administer injectable medications in a manner that maximally enhances health benefits for the patient.

- The student shows knowledge of appropriate routes of injection for commonly used medications as well as differences among parenteral administration routes regarding relative rates of absorption, onset of effect, and duration of effect.
- The student demonstrates understanding of how the characteristics (such as temperament) and clinical status (such as a seizing patient) of an individual patient determine how to appropriately administer injectable medications.
- The student displays knowledge of potential complications associated with common parenteral administration routes.
- The student demonstrates appreciation of the importance of accurately identifying and selecting correct medications and of checking the label at least three times to assure selection of the correct drug, dosage concentration, administration route, and so on.
- The student displays understanding of the importance of checking the bottle for cracks, expiration dates, reconstitution dates, foreign matter, color changes, precipitation, and other signs of nonviability.
- The student shows knowledge of how to use correct aseptic technique.

47) **The student properly administers subcutaneous injections to dogs, cats, and ruminants.**
- The student demonstrates the ability to determine proper injection sites in common domestic species.
- The student appropriately prepares the site for injection.
- The student selects the appropriate size/gauge syringe and needle.

- The student properly holds the syringe and inserts the needle with the bevel up at the correct angle and depth.
- The student aspirates the syringe to check for blood, air, and/or improper placement.
- The student administers the correct dose of the appropriate medication, withdraws the needle, and gently massages the injection site.
- The student properly disposes of the syringe and needle.

48) **The student properly administers intramuscular injections to dogs, cats, and horses/ponies/donkeys/mules.**
- Using appropriate landmarks, the student demonstrates the ability to determine proper injection sites in common domestic species.
- The student appropriately prepares the site for injection.
- The student selects the appropriate size/gauge syringe and needle.
- The student properly holds the syringe and inserts the needle at the correct angle and depth.
- The student aspirates the syringe to check for blood, air, and/or improper placement.
- The student administers the correct dose of the appropriate medication, withdraws the needle, and gently massages the injection site.
- The student properly disposes of the syringe and needle.

49) **The student correctly administers direct-bolus, intravenous injections to dogs, cats, ruminants, and horses/ponies/donkeys/mules.**
- The student demonstrates the ability to identify proper injection sites in common domestic species.
- The student accurately palpates and isolates the vein for injection.
- The student appropriately prepares the site for injection, using an assistant or a tourniquet to "raise" and stabilize the vein.

- The student properly holds the syringe and inserts the needle, bevel up, into the vein at the correct angle, aspirating the syringe to check for blood in the hub.
- When administering medications with a butterfly catheter, the student correctly holds the catheter and inserts the needle, bevel up, into the vein at a correct angle, allowing the blood to fill the tubing.
- The student removes the tourniquet or has the assistant release pressure on the vein at the appropriate time.
- The student administers a correct dose of the right medication, at an appropriate administration rate (time interval), while making certain that the needle is properly stabilized in the vein and that the entire dose is given intravenously, making certain not to administer any air into the patient.
- When using a butterfly catheter, the student appropriately flushes the catheter following the injection of medication to ensure delivery of the entire volume of medication, making certain not to inject any air into the patient.
- The student withdraws the needle and applies appropriate pressure or appropriately places bandage to the venipuncture site to stop bleeding.

50) **The student considers the individual patient's characteristics and physical status when administering non-injectable medications in order to provide maximal benefits with minimal risk and stress to the patient.**
  - The student displays knowledge of various enteral administration routes and of potential complications associated with each.
  - The student explains behavior characteristics and disease states that may make certain enteral routes of administration inappropriate.

- The student demonstrates appreciation of the importance of accurately identifying and selecting correct medications and of checking the label at least three times to assure selection of the correct drug, dosage concentration, administration route, and so on.
- The student displays understanding of the importance of checking the bottle for cracks, expiration dates, reconstitution dates, foreign matter, color changes, precipitation, and other signs of nonviability.

51) **The student demonstrates the ability to properly utilize a balling gun to administer medications to ruminants.**
  - The student demonstrates knowledge of pertinent oral and pharyngeal anatomy.
  - The student appropriately restrains the animal and demonstrates awareness of safety protocols.
  - The student demonstrates proper use of the balling gun.
  - The student monitors the patient to be certain the medication is properly received.

52) **The student displays the ability to correctly utilize a dose syringe to administer medications to ruminants and horses/ponies/donkeys/mules.**
  - The student appropriately restrains the animal and demonstrates awareness of safety protocols.
  - The student demonstrates the ability to administer small volumes of liquid, using a dose syringe.
  - The student monitors the patient to be certain the medication is properly received.

53) **The student properly hand-pills dogs and cats.**
  - The student understands contraindications to and potential complications of oral administration of medications.
  - The student employs proper technique for hand-pilling the dog, while maintaining safe restraint.

- The student employs proper technique for hand-pilling the cat, while maintaining safe restraint.
- The student administers water via syringe following the oral administration of dry drugs to assist in the movement of the drug through the esophagus and into the stomach as well as to avoid esophageal injury/stricture.
- The student monitors the animal to make certain the medication was properly received.

54) **The student correctly administers topical, otic, and ophthalmic medications.**
- The student describes precautions for handling and safety when administering topical, otic, and ophthalmic medications.
- For topical medications, the student clips and cleanses the affected area as needed.
- Wearing gloves, the student applies the proper amount of topical medication in the appropriate area as prescribed.
- The student demonstrates knowledge of the anatomy of the ear canal and the importance of ensuring that the tympanic membrane is intact prior to the administration of otic medications.
- For otic medications, the student cleans the ear prior to administration of medication, when appropriate, to remove debris in order to increase effectiveness. Prior to administration, the student makes certain that the medication is the correct prescribed otic medication. To administer otic medications, the student correctly grasps the pinna and pulls upward and slightly laterally in order to straighten the ear canal when administering medication. After administering otic medication, the student massages the base of the ear canal to ensure distribution of the medication.
- Prior to administration, the student makes certain that the medication is the correct prescribed ophthalmic medication.
- To administer ophthalmic medications, the student properly restrains the animal's head and, keeping the head stable, opens the eyelid.
- The student properly administers ocular drops/ointment, ensuring that the applicator tip does not touch the eye and remains sterile.
- The student makes certain that the animal does not rub its eye with its paws or rub its eye against any object immediately post-treatment.
- When necessary, the student applies an e-collar to prevent the animal from reaching the affected area.

55) **The student participates in the proper administration of enemas.**
- The student demonstrates knowledge of the pertinent anatomy as well as disease states that may require the administration of an enema.
- The student demonstrates understanding of potential complications of administering enemas, such as damage to rectal mucosa, transmission of infection, and so on.
- The student shows awareness that enemas should be performed only when indicated, due to their potential risks.
- The student shows understanding of the advantages and potential adverse effects of different enema solutions.
- The student prepares all equipment in advance, making certain enema solutions are at or near body temperature.
- When administering enemas to cats, the student makes certain that a clean litter box is waiting in the cage.
- The student describes proper restraint of the animal for administration of an enema.
- The student explains the proper procedure for administration of enemas.
- The student displays appreciation of the need to quickly move the animal to a run/cage or outdoors immediately after enema administration in order to allow bowel evacuation.
- The student shows appreciation of the importance of cleaning and drying the

animal's hindquarters and placing the animal in a clean run/cage after bowel evacuation.

56) **The student participates in the correct placement of a stomach tube in small animals.**

- The student demonstrates knowledge of pertinent anatomy as well as disease states that may require the placement of a stomach tube.
- The student demonstrates awareness of potential complications of stomach tube placement in small animals.
- The student displays knowledge of various types of stomach tubes, such as nasogastric and orogastric, and their appropriate indications.
- The student describes how to select an appropriate size (diameter and length) tube based on the patient's size and the purpose of the stomach tube.
- The student explains proper techniques for stomach tube placement including why checking proper tube placement is essential.
- The student shows knowledge of how to check for proper stomach tube placement prior to the administration of any substance that may be harmful to the respiratory tract.

57) **The student correctly obtains and microscopically evaluates skin scrapings.**

- The student displays knowledge of the dermatologic disease states that can be diagnosed with a skin scrape.
- The student correctly identifies the lesion to be scraped. The student describes proper techniques for superficial and deep skin scrapings and the indications for each.
- The student properly performs the skin scraping.
- The student transfers collected hair and epithelial debris to a glass slide by scraping the material against the edge of the slide and then mixes the collected material with the mineral oil.

- The student properly uses the microscope to examine and correctly evaluate the collected material, and appropriately records the results in the animal's medical record.

58) **The student properly administers fluids by the subcutaneous route.**

- The student demonstrates understanding of the pertinent anatomy.
- The student is able to differentiate types of fluids that may be administered subcutaneously from those that should not.
- The student displays understanding of how subcutaneous fluids are absorbed, the amount of fluid that can be safely administered by the subcutaneous route, and potential complications associated with the subcutaneous administration of fluids.
- The student properly prepares all needed equipment in advance, including the correct fluid bag, the appropriate administration set, and correct needle gauge, avoiding contamination. The student inspects the fluid bag for expiration date, integrity of sterile packaging, discoloration, cloudiness, and so on. If appropriate, the student pre-warms the fluids to body temperature, making certain the fluid temperature does not exceed body temperature.
- The student appropriately restrains the animal.
- The student properly identifies and prepares the administration site.
- Using correct technique, the student administers the correct volume of fluids at an appropriate flow rate, monitoring for patency of the administration set and the correct placement of the needle. The student clamps off the tubing and withdraws the needle, then applies pressure to the injection site.
- The student displays the ability to explain and demonstrate to an owner how to properly and safely administer subcutaneous fluids, how they are absorbed, and their benefits to the

animal. The student demonstrates the ability to properly educate clients as to the safe disposal of needles and potential complications of subcutaneous fluid administration.

59) **The student properly places intravenous catheters into the cephalic and saphenous veins.**

- The student demonstrates knowledge of the pertinent anatomy, relative advantages and disadvantages of each site, and the potential complications associated with catheterization of each site.
- The student displays knowledge of the indications for use, benefits, and limitations of each catheter type.
- The student prepares, in advance, all necessary equipment, such as sterile gloves, scrub solution, alcohol, gauze pads, bandage material, tape, appropriate size and type of catheter, T-connector or injection cap, saline or heparinized saline flushes, empty syringes, blood tubes, clippers, and so on.
- The student has the assistant appropriately position and restrain the animal.
- With gloved hands, the student aseptically prepares the site. The student correctly isolates, palpates, raises, and stabilizes the vein. Wearing sterile gloves and maintaining aseptic technique, the student correctly and successfully places the catheter in the vein. The student verifies proper placement and patency of the catheter.
- The student properly secures the catheter with tape in a way that minimizes trauma to the vein.
- The student appropriately applies the bandage in a manner that secures placement of the catheter, permits access to the catheter for blood sampling; administration of fluids or medication; and minimizes potential complications as well as discomfort to the patient.

60) **The student properly cares for and attentively monitors intravenous catheters.**

- The student displays knowledge of complications associated with indwelling intravenous catheters.
- When indicated, the student flushes indwelling catheters (e.g., with sterile saline solution), checking the patency and integrity of the catheter.
- At appropriate intervals, the student checks for signs of inflammation, infection, swelling, or patient discomfort; the student also checks the bandage for slippage, moisture, cleanliness, or signs of patient discomfort.
- The student appropriately changes the catheter and/or bandage when necessary.

61) **The student accurately calculates fluid infusion rates and explains how to monitor fluid administration to ensure correct administration rates.**

- The student defines the terms *hydration deficit, maintenance requirements,* and *ongoing losses,* and demonstrates understanding of the clinical implications of each.
- The student displays knowledge of various crystalloid solutions, including which are balanced versus non-balanced solutions and which are isotonic, hypotonic, or hypertonic. The student shows awareness of proper indications and major contraindications for various types of crystalloid solutions, as well as any special requirements for their administration.
- The student displays knowledge of various colloids, including natural and synthetic, their proper indications, and any special requirements for their administration.
- The student accurately calculates fluid requirements, considering hydration deficits, maintenance requirements, and ongoing losses.
- The student accurately calculates appropriate fluid infusion rates.
- The student displays understanding of how to administer fluids at appropriate

rates and how to monitor to ensure that the fluid is flowing freely at the correct rate.

- The student demonstrates knowledge of common additives, such as KCl solution, vitamin B complex, and 50% dextrose solution.
- The student correctly calculates the volume of common additives and appropriately adds it to the fluids.
- The student shows understanding of the importance of correctly labeling fluid bags to indicate additives per liter bag of fluids, the date of preparation, and their initials.
- The student displays knowledge of common problems that can occur with fluid administration, such as a kink in the administration set, a clot in the catheter, a malfunction of the infusion pump, and so on, and explains how to correct them.

62) **The student demonstrates knowledge of how to correctly monitor and evaluate the hydration status of patients.**

- The student demonstrates knowledge of body fluid compartments. The student distinguishes classical signs associated with fluid losses from each body fluid compartment.
- The student explains how to evaluate patient hydration status qualitatively by assessment of skin turgor, moistness of mucous membranes, positioning of the eye within its socket, thoracic auscultation, pulse rate and strength, and patient demeanor. In animals receiving subcutaneous fluids, the student evaluates ventral or dependent anatomic areas to assess fluid absorption.
- The student describes how to evaluate patient hydration status quantitatively by accurate measurement of body weight (using same scale each time), PCV, plasma proteins, and urine specific gravity (and urine output, if necessary).

- The student displays understanding of central venous pressure (CVP) and its role in assessing hydration status.
- The student demonstrates knowledge of how to recognize signs of overhydration by evaluation of lung sounds, heart rate, respiratory rate, conjunctiva, the presence of peripheral edema or serous nasal discharge, bounding pulses, and/or increased urination.

63) **The student demonstrates familiarity with various fluid delivery systems.**

- The student shows knowledge of and correctly identifies various fluid delivery systems, such as macrodrip and microdrip administration sets, volume control systems (Buretrol® sets), secondary administration sets, and extension sets.
- The student demonstrates understanding of how to operate infusion pumps correctly as well as potential causes of malfunction and how to troubleshoot problems appropriately.
- The student displays knowledge of how to correctly administer fluids without a fluid pump. For example, how to establish and maintain the appropriate drip rate.

64) **The student properly applies and removes bandages and splints.**

- The student demonstrates understanding of the need to bandage wounds, fractures, catheter sites, and so on. The student demonstrates knowledge of indications for different bandage types.
- The student displays knowledge of different types of primary bandaging materials, such as paraffin gauze, perforated film dressing, foam dressing, and hydrocolloids, and their clinical application on the wound.
- The student correctly applies bandages, including, but not limited to, the following steps: the student applies stirrups, selects appropriate primary, secondary, and tertiary layers and applies an appropriate protective layer.

- The student demonstrates an understanding of appropriate uses of different types/sizes of splints and correctly applies them.
- The student demonstrates knowledge of specialized bandages appropriate to specific situations, including, but not limited to, Robert Jones bandages, modified Robert Jones bandages, chest or abdominal bandages, Velpeau slings, and Ehmer slings.
- The student explains appropriate bandage care and how to recognize and address complications.
- The student correctly and safely removes bandages and splints.

65) **The student displays knowledge of appropriate care of wounds and abscesses.**
   - The student demonstrates knowledge of appropriate wound management and abscess care, including the immediate care of the wound or abscess; lavage and debridement; and, based on the individual wound, methods of wound closure and their appropriate uses.
   - The student demonstrates understanding of the appropriate uses of topical and systemic therapeutics for wounds and abscesses.
   - The student displays understanding of the importance of appropriately using devices such as E-collars or recovery suits to protect the wound or abscess from self-inflicted trauma (such as licking or scratching).

66) **The student demonstrates the ability to explain proper care of the recumbent patient.**
   - The student demonstrates understanding of basic requirements for care of recumbent patients, including, but not limited to, proper bedding, carefully turning the patient to avoid hypostatic congestion and decubitus, passive range of motion (PROM) to reduce muscle atrophy and maintain joint mobility, massage therapy

to prevent edema in dependent limbs, monitoring of urine/stool output, vital signs, nutritional requirements, and mental stimulation.
   - The student displays appreciation of the importance of keeping the recumbent patient clean and dry.

67) **The student participates in collecting and crossmatch testing blood for transfusion.**
   - The student displays knowledge of canine and feline blood types.
   - The student shows understanding of the importance of crossmatch testing.
   - The student demonstrates knowledge of potential complications of incompatible blood transfusions.
   - The student correctly identifies and labels blood collection tubes for recipient and donor blood samples.
   - The student participates in properly performing crossmatch testing.
   - The student correctly identifies the presence or absence of agglutination. The student accurately interprets test results and correctly chooses an appropriate donor.

68) **The student demonstrates knowledge of how to properly stock and maintain an emergency crash cart.**
   - The student shows appreciation of the importance of preparing and maintaining an emergency crash cart.
   - The student displays knowledge of the essential components of a well-stocked, mobile emergency crash cart.
   - The student describes how to properly maintain a well-organized, mobile emergency crash cart.
   - The student demonstrates familiarity with all equipment needed to perform successful cardiopulmonary resuscitation (CPR) and explains how to regularly perform necessary equipment maintenance.
   - The student demonstrates awareness of the uses, indications, major contraindications, common adverse effects, and

appropriate administration routes of commonly used emergency drugs.

69) **The student demonstrates competence in administering first aid and cardiopulmonary resuscitation (CPR).**

- The student demonstrates knowledge of safety protocols for administering first aid to patients. For example, injured animals should be appropriately restrained because they may become aggressive due to fear and pain.
- The student displays knowledge of how to safely transport an injured animal, demonstrating understanding of the importance of minimizing movement.
- The student shows knowledge of the proper techniques for minimizing hemorrhage.
- The student demonstrates knowledge of the proper techniques for stabilizing fractures.
- The student displays knowledge of how to triage patients for assessment by the veterinarian.
- The student demonstrates the ability to accurately identify patients most at risk for respiratory and/or cardiopulmonary arrest. The student shows knowledge of disease processes and/or drugs (including anesthetic and analgesic agents) that may predispose animals to respiratory and/or cardiopulmonary arrest.
- The student demonstrates appreciation of the importance of recognizing and treating abnormalities before arrest occurs (i.e., preventing arrest is better than treating arrest).
- The student shows understanding of the fact that preparedness and early recognition increase the chance of successful CPR.
- The student shows understanding of the importance of training and regularly practicing CPR with all available staff members.
- The student demonstrates knowledge of normal vital signs. The student recognizes normal cardiac rhythms and

demonstrates the ability to differentiate normal from abnormal. The student recognizes normal respiratory rates, depths, and patterns and demonstrates the ability to differentiate normal from abnormal.

- The student displays understanding of the importance of closely monitoring vital signs in all patients at risk for respiratory and/or cardiopulmonary arrest. In patients under general anesthesia, the student shows understanding of the importance of closely observing vital signs and anesthetic monitoring equipment, as well as carefully and frequently evaluating respiratory function (adequacy of oxygenation and ventilation), circulatory function, and the degree of central nervous system (CNS) depression (decreases in muscle tone and CNS reflexes).
- The student demonstrates knowledge of how to promptly recognize signs of impending cardiopulmonary arrest (CPA), including significant, abnormal changes in respiratory frequency, character (depth and/or pattern), or sound (agonal gasps); weak and/or significantly abnormal pulses; arrhythmias and/or changes in heart sounds; significant changes in body temperature and/or blood pressure; and/or abnormal mucous membrane color. In patients under general anesthesia, the student also shows knowledge of other indicators of impending arrest, including, but not limited to, significant abnormalities in electrocardiogram (ECG), SpO_2, pH, PaO_2, PvO_2, $ETCO_2$, and/or severe loss of muscle tone and CNS reflexes.
- The student exhibits knowledge of how to promptly recognize signs of cardiopulmonary arrest, including unconsciousness; absence of heart sounds and palpable pulses; absence of ventilatory efforts and breath sounds (agonal gasps may be heard); cyanotic, gray, or white mucous membranes; and dilated pupils

Berg, M. and Eliason, J. (2022). Role of the veterinary technicians and hygienists in veterinary dentistry and oral surgery. *Vet Clin Small Anim* 52: 49–66, https://doi.org/10.1016/j.cvsm.2021.09.007.

Douglas, D., Buell, L. J., and Schenkel, L. E. (2017). Laboratory animal care and procedures. In *Assessing Essential Skills of Veterinary Technology Students*, 3rd e. (ed. L. J. Buell, L. E. Schenkel, and S. Timperman), 9–23. Ames: John Wiley & Sons, Inc.

Fletcher, D., Boller, M., Brainard, B., Haskins, S., Hopper, K., McMichael, M., Smarick, S. (2012, June). RECOVER evidence and knowledge gap analysis on veterinary CPR. Part 7: Clinical guidelines. *J Vet Emerg Crit Care* 22 (Supplement 1), S103–S131.

Holstrom, S. E. (2019). *Veterinary Dentistry a Team Approach* (3rd e.) (pp. 153–198). St. Louis: Elsevier.

Martin, D. and Martin, K. (2022). FAS (FEAR, ANXIETY & STRESS) SCALE. https://www.edinburghpets.com/wp-content/uploads/2023/11/FAS-Scale_final-2022-2.pdf.

Monteiro, B. P., Lascelles, B. D. X., Murrell, J., Robertson, S., Steagall, P. V. M., and Wright, B. (2022). *2022* WSAVA guidelines for the recognition, assessment and treatment of pain. Retrieved October 4, 2023, from https://onlinelibrary.wiley.com/.

Université de Montréal (2019). *Feline Grimace Scale©*. Retrieved October 4, 2023, from https://www.felinegrimacescale.com.

4

Anesthesia
Lisa E. Schenkel, DVM, CCRT, CVMA, Sandra Lynn Bertholf, MS, LVT, and Amanda Colón, DVM

4.1 Perioperative Management of the Veterinary Patient

1) **The student demonstrates the ability to work with the veterinarian to accurately evaluate the physical status and anesthetic risk of individual patients.**
   - The student displays understanding that general anesthesia is an inherently compromised state that is produced by drugs that depress the central nervous system (CNS). As such, general anesthesia carries risks of complications, primarily due to adverse physiologic changes to respiratory system, cardiovascular system, and central nervous system function.
   - The student shows knowledge of the American Society of Anesthesiologists (ASA) classification of patient physical status (Brodbelt, Flaherty, and Pettifer, 2015).
   - The student demonstrates understanding that the patient's potential for survival of general anesthesia is, in part, determined by the individual animal's physical status.
   - The student shows awareness that the animal's physical status is determined by signalment, patient history, physical examination, diagnostic tests, and the procedure to be performed.

- The student demonstrates understanding that the animal's anesthetic risk often is affected by signalment (species, breed, age, weight, reproductive status, temperament, etc.). For example, brachycephalic breeds often have partially obstructed airways due to structural abnormalities. Neonatal animals are prone to hypothermia, dehydration, and hypoglycemia, as well as a decreased ability to biotransform drugs due to immature liver function. Geriatric animals may be less able to biotransform and excrete drugs due to decreased liver and/or kidney function. The student shows knowledge that the animal's weight must be accurate because it determines drug dosages, fluid administration rates, and, often, the type of anesthetic system used (rebreathing vs non-rebreathing).
- The student appropriately works with the veterinarian to gather as much accurate information as possible on the patient relevant to anesthesia prior to and during the pre-anesthetic period.

2) **Based on the individual patient's physical status, anesthetic risk, and type of procedure, the student demonstrates the ability to work with the veterinarian to tailor anesthetic and analgesic**

Assessing Essential Skills of Veterinary Technology Students, Fourth Edition. Edited by Lisa E. Schenkel, Amanda Colón, Sandra Lynn Bertholf, Sabrina Timperman, and Laurie J. Buell.
Companion website: www.wiley.com/go/Schenkel/AssessingEssentialSkillsofVeterinaryTechnologyStudents4e

regimens to meet the needs of the individual patient with the goals of maximizing safety, while minimizing and/or preventing nociception and pain.

- The student accurately defines the terms *anesthesia, general anesthesia, surgical anesthesia, balanced (multimodal) anesthesia, local anesthesia, regional anesthesia, neuroleptic anesthesia,* and *dissociative anesthesia.* The student demonstrates understanding of the appropriate clinical applications of each.
- The student displays understanding of the pre-anesthetic period as the time to anticipate potential complications, attempt to optimize the animal's condition and take proactive steps to prevent complications from arising. For example, the student demonstrates awareness that brachycephalic breeds generally need very rapid anesthetic induction, intubation, and anesthetic recovery (to maintain patent airways), and very close monitoring following extubation. As another example, the student takes special care to closely monitor the body temperature of neonates and keep them warm, preparing appropriate warming devices, such as hot water circulating blankets, Bair huggers® and/or Hot Dog® patient warming systems. Even in emergency procedures, the student displays awareness that, if time allows, all steps should be taken to correct and stabilize the following conditions prior to anesthetic induction: dehydration, hypovolemia, hypotension, anemia, hypoproteinemia, cardiac dysfunction, respiratory distress, renal dysfunction, clotting defects, and hyperthermia or hypothermia.
- Following the veterinarian's orders, during the pre-anesthetic period, the student secures venous access to administer injectable anesthetic and analgesic drugs and to administer fluids to prevent and/or treat dehydration and/or hypotension, as well as to speed the rate of drug elimination. In addition, securing venous access during the pre-anesthetic period provides an administration route for emergency drugs, if needed.
- Following the veterinarian's orders, the student fasts patients and withholds water for the appropriate time periods prior to anesthetic induction, if proper for the individual patient. The student displays awareness that birds, neonates, and exotic animals may be fasted for very short periods or not at all due to their tendency to become hypoglycemic. The student also displays awareness that fasting species that are hind-gut fermenters, such as rabbits and guinea pigs, can lead to gastrointestinal ileus.
- The student displays awareness that only the veterinarian may prescribe anesthetic agents, doses, and routes of administration. In addition, the student shows understanding that it is the technician's/technologist's duty to make appropriate suggestions and communicate pertinent observations to the supervising veterinarian.
- The student displays awareness that no pre-anesthetic, anesthetic or analgesic agent is free from adverse effects and that no single agent is safe for all animals. The student, therefore, demonstrates understanding that determination of pre-anesthetic, anesthetic and analgesic protocols should be tailored to the individual patient based on patient's signalment, physical status, co-morbidities, type and duration of procedure, existing and anticipated pain level, inpatient versus outpatient, elective versus emergency procedures, and the veterinarian's and technician's/technologist's experience.

3) **The student accurately calculates dosages of agents administered during the peri-anesthetic period.**

- During the pre-anesthetic period (on the day of the procedure), the student accurately weighs the patient and records the weight in the patient's record.

- The student correctly calculates doses of anesthetic and analgesic drugs based on the patient's weight, when appropriate.
  a) The student shows awareness that, in overweight animals, doses of anesthetic-related drugs should be calculated based on lean body weight, rather than actual body weight.
  b) The student displays awareness that doses of anesthetic-related drugs should be reduced in emaciated animals.
- The student correctly prepares and accurately measures doses of enterally and parenterally administered anesthetic and analgesic agents.
- The student correctly documents calculated doses in patient medical records.
  a) The student accurately records the calculated doses of drugs in correct units of measure, for example, in grams (g), milligrams (mg), micrograms (mcg), International Units (IU), or milliequivalents (mEq).
  b) The student displays awareness that the dosage strength of the drug (e.g., mg/ml, mg/tab) must be included when recording the dosage form of the drug (e.g., number of oral tablets or number of ml of an injectable solution).
  c) For agents administered "to effect," the student uses "drawn/given" method, writing on the patient's record both the amount of drug drawn up and the amount actually administered. For controlled drugs, the student uses the "drawn/given" method in the controlled substances log.

4) **The student demonstrates the ability to properly administer pre-anesthetic, anesthetic, and analgesic agents by appropriate routes, including anesthetic induction by injectable agents, as well as the administration of anesthetic gases and oxygen by mask and endotracheal tube.**
- The student demonstrates basic understanding of appropriate uses, major

contraindications, common adverse effects, and appropriate routes and methods of administration for commonly used, injectable anesthetic and pre-anesthetic agents, and their reversal agents, where applicable.
- The student demonstrates basic understanding of properties, appropriate uses, major contraindications, and common adverse effects of inhalant anesthetic agents, such as isoflurane and sevoflurane.
- The student demonstrates understanding of relative advantages and disadvantages of the various methods of anesthetic induction and utilizes each appropriately. The student displays awareness that mask inductions permit anesthetic induction without IV access and may be warranted in individual cases. The student displays knowledge of disadvantages associated with mask inductions, including but not limited to: lack of airway control, increased dead space, prolonged Stage II (compared with intravenously administered induction agents), increased patient stress and increased atmospheric pollution with anesthetic gas.
- The student demonstrates the ability to properly administer injectable anesthetic-related drugs by bolus and/or constant rate infusion.
- The student properly administers inhalant anesthetic agents by mask and endotracheal tube.
- The student correctly records the dose as well as the time and route of administration of anesthetic-related agents used in the patient's anesthetic record.

5) **The student demonstrates the ability to endotracheally intubate patients correctly and safely.**
- The student displays knowledge of the relevant anatomy to correctly and safely place an endotracheal tube.
- The student demonstrates knowledge of the advantages of endotracheal intubation, such as reducing dead space,

decreasing exposure of personnel to waste gases, maintaining a patent airway, allowing assisted or controlled ventilation, and decreasing risk of aspiration of vomitus, saliva, and/or blood (when the cuff is inflated).

- The student displays understanding of the potential complications of overly aggressive intubation or overinflation of the cuff, including but not limited to endotracheal inflammation, necrosis, or tracheal rupture; trauma to the soft palate, pharynx or larynx; stimulation of the vagus nerve, potentially leading to bradycardia or other cardiac dysrhythmias; and/or damage to the recurrent laryngeal nerve, potentially leading to laryngeal paralysis and/or bradycardia. The student shows awareness of the need to avoid laryngeal trauma, particularly in cats, to avoid laryngospasm and excessive mucous secretion.
- The student demonstrates awareness that underinflation of the cuff dilutes the percentage of inhalant anesthetic reaching the gas exchange portion of the lungs, as well as increasing the risk of aspiration.
- The student selects the appropriate size and diameter endotracheal (ET) tube. The student demonstrates awareness that the distal end of tube should not extend beyond the level of thoracic inlet.
  a) The student pre-measures the distance from incisors to the cervical trachea near the thoracic inlet.
  b) To minimize mechanical dead space, the student avoids use of an overly long ET tube, making certain the connector is very near the incisors.
  c) The student demonstrates understanding that too narrow a diameter or too long an ET tube increases resistance to breathing.
- The student accurately identifies the anesthetic depth (stage and plane of anesthesia) at which intubation is appropriate. For example, the student shows

awareness that laryngospasm may result when intubation is attempted in a cat at too light an anesthetic plane.

- In placing the ET tube, the student carefully avoids overly aggressive intubation, underinflation, and overinflation of the cuff.
- The student checks to ensure proper placement of the ET tube by ausculting the lungs and ensuring that breath sounds are present in all lung fields. The student shows awareness that proper ET tube placement also can be confirmed by capnography.
- The student secures the ET tube in place in a manner suitable for the species and type of procedure.
- The student regularly monitors for proper cuff inflation, obstruction, or movement of the ET tube. The student deflates the cuff prior to repositioning or removing the ET tube.
- The student safely extubates the patient at the appropriate time (generally when oral and pharyngeal reflexes have returned) to avoid chewing on the tube by the patient.
- The student records the time of intubation and extubation in the patient's anesthesia record.

6) **Based on observation of clinical signs and the correct use of monitoring equipment, the student demonstrates the ability to accurately monitor the patient's status throughout all stages of the procedure.**

- The student demonstrates understanding of the essential components of anesthesia, including but not limited to the preanesthetic period, anesthetic induction, maintenance, and recovery; anesthetic monitoring; and pain assessment and pain management.
- The student shows awareness of the patient's ongoing status before, during, and after anesthesia to provide for adequate anesthesia, analgesia, and safe

recovery. The student does not leave the animal unobserved during the peri-anesthetic and anesthetic periods, including following administration of pre-anesthetic medications as well as during anesthetic recovery, both before and after extubation.

- The student shows understanding that the physiologic status of the anesthetized patient is evaluated through assessment of respiratory, cardiovascular, and central nervous system function.
  a) The student demonstrates knowledge of values for vital signs, neuromuscular signs (degree of muscle tone), and CNS reflexes (e.g., swallowing, palpebral, pedal, corneal) associated with each phase of central nervous system (CNS) depression (and/or each stage of anesthesia).
  b) The student shows familiarity with acceptable values for vital signs, neuromuscular signs, and CNS reflexes in awake and recovering animals.
- The student demonstrates understanding that, for American Society of Anesthesiologists (ASA) Status I or II patients, a veterinarian or veterinary technician/technologist should be continuously present with and focused on assessing the patient's respiratory, cardiovascular, and CNS function. The student shows awareness that, if this is not possible, patient status should be monitored a minimum of every five minutes during anesthesia and throughout the recovery period (American College of Veterinary Anesthesiologists, 2009).
- The student shows understanding that, for ASA Status III, IV, or V patients, or for any horse anesthetized with an inhalant anesthetic, or for any horse anesthetized for longer than 45 minutes, a veterinarian or veterinary technician/technologist should be continuously present with the patient and focused on assessing the patient's respiratory, cardiovascular, and

CNS function, during anesthesia and throughout the recovery period (American College of Veterinary Anesthesiologists, 2009).

- The student demonstrates understanding of the importance of maintaining an anesthetic record for each patient, both as legal documentation of significant events and to facilitate identification of trends in monitored values, thereby allowing early recognition of potential complications.
- The student accurately records parameters in the anesthetic record a minimum of every five minutes.
- The student displays awareness that monitoring equipment is not a reliable replacement for the technician's/technologist's eyes, ears, and hands. As much as is practical, the student uses their senses to monitor vital signs, muscle tone, and reflexes, including, but not limited to: direct palpation of pulse rate and strength; auscultation of the chest with a stethoscope for heart rate and rhythm and the presence of abnormal respiratory sounds; observation of the animal's chest and reservoir bag for respiratory rate and depth; monitoring capillary refill time, mucous membrane color, and body temperature; and checking muscle tone and reflexes to help assess the level of CNS depression. The student displays knowledge of acceptable values for all parameters, both awake and under anesthesia.
- The student uses appropriate monitoring equipment to aid in assessing patient status at all times during and following the procedure. The student displays the ability to use a stethoscope and differentiate normal from abnormal heart sounds; use a blood pressure monitor and differentiate acceptable arterial blood pressures from hypo- or hypertension; and use an electrocardiograph and differentiate normal from abnormal ECGs. The student demonstrates the ability to use a pulse

oximeter and a capnometer/capnograph to assess the adequacy of oxygenation and ventilation.

7) **The student demonstrates understanding of how to assess the patient for evidence of nociception and/or pain, administer analgesic therapy properly and in accordance with the veterinarian's orders, and carefully monitor the efficacy of analgesic therapy.**

- The student displays understanding of the importance of the technician/technologist's role in assessing pain and conveying the assessment to the veterinarian so that an appropriate and effective pain management protocol can be implemented and sustained.
- The student demonstrates familiarity with the difference between physiologic and pathologic pain.
- The student correctly defines terms such as *visceral pain, deep somatic pain, superficial somatic pain, adaptive pain, maladaptive pain, neuropathic pain,* and *inflammatory pain.*
- The student demonstrates knowledge of the physiological process of nociception and pain perception:
  a) The student correctly explains the physiological events leading to central and peripheral sensitization.
  b) The student accurately describes the terms *hyperalgesia* and *allodynia.*
  c) The student explains the clinical implications of maladaptive pain in developing effective pain management protocols.
- The student displays knowledge of physiological signs of pain resulting from reflex ventilatory, cardiovascular, and hormonal responses to nociception. The student demonstrates awareness that objective signs of pain, including increases in respiratory rate, heart rate, arterial blood pressure, catecholamine, and cortisol levels, are not necessarily correlated with the intensity of pain

sensation (Buell, 1999; Wiese and Yaksh, 2015; Muir III, 2015).

- The student demonstrates knowledge of obvious behaviors associated with pain, such as vocalization, resentment of palpation, trembling, reluctance to move or bear weight, self-mutilation, hunched-up posture, and so on. The student demonstrates awareness that vocalization is not necessarily correlated with pain intensity, lack of obvious pain behaviors does not indicate lack of pain, and behavioral signs of pain may be very subtle, making very close monitoring essential (Wiese, 2015).
- The student demonstrates knowledge of normal behaviors characteristic of particular species and breeds. The student also shows awareness of behaviors induced by pain in particular species and breeds. For example, lack of grooming or overgrooming in a specific area may be an indication of pain in cats, while kicking at the abdomen may be sign of pain in horses.
- The student shows awareness that deviation from the individual animal's normal behaviors may be evidence of pain (e.g., inability to sleep, anorexia, depression, apprehensiveness, or a normally friendly animal behaving aggressively or unwilling to interact) (Wiese, 2015).
- The student demonstrates knowledge of how the effects of drugs, such as tranquilizers and anesthetic agents, can interfere with accurate pain assessment. For example, an animal who has been sedated may not exhibit pain-induced behaviors but still be experiencing significant pain.
- The student displays knowledge of potentially detrimental physiological effects of pain, including diminished wound healing, impaired immune system function, and the release of proinflammatory cytokines (Wiese and Yaksh, 2015).
- The student demonstrates awareness that the effects of not treating pain often are

more deleterious than the potential adverse effects associated with recommended dosages of analgesic drugs (Wiese, Muir III, and Wittum, 2005).

- The student displays awareness that, as an adjunct to thorough patient evaluation, appropriate use of pain scales is necessary in ensuring that pain is properly assessed and treated.

- The student demonstrates understanding of how to judge the efficacy of pain therapy in the individual animal, based on reduction of behaviors associated with pain, as well as return to more normal behavior for the individual animal.

- The student shows understanding of the concepts of analgesia, preemptive analgesia, multimodal analgesia, and balanced analgesia.

- The student demonstrates basic understanding of the appropriate uses, major contraindications, common adverse effects, and appropriate routes and methods of administration for commonly used analgesic agents. These may include, but are not limited to, opioid analgesic agents (and their reversal agents), non-steroidal anti-inflammatory agents, NMDA-receptor antagonists (such as ketamine), alpha$_2$ agonists (and their reversal agents), and local anesthetic agents.

- The student displays knowledge of how to implement appropriate pain management protocols, while continuing to monitor the patient's ongoing status. The student demonstrates knowledge that any animal given analgesic agents must be closely monitored for adverse effects in the pre-anesthetic period, the anesthetic period, and the entire recovery period.

8) **The student demonstrates knowledge of how to detect anesthetic complications and respond to them quickly and appropriately.**
   - The student shows understanding of the importance of being proactive in managing the anesthetized patient by anticipating likely complications and taking appropriate steps to avoid them.

- The student demonstrates knowledge of how to take steps to avoid and closely monitor for the presence of abnormalities, potential complications, and/or clinically significant changes in patient status that may arise during the anesthetic and/or peri-anesthetic period.

- The student displays awareness of the need to immediately inform the supervisor/veterinarian of any anesthetic complications.

- The student demonstrates knowledge of how to address complications rapidly and appropriately.

- The student displays understanding of how to rapidly recognize and respond to respiratory complications. For example, the student shows awareness of an SpO$_2$ of <95% as evidence of hypoxemia. The student displays knowledge of common causes of hypoxemia during anesthesia, including, but not limited to, inadequate O$_2$ flow, loss of airway, or obstruction of the breathing circuit. The student demonstrates knowledge of malfunctions in the oxygen supply, anesthetic machine, ET tube and/or breathing circuit that may lead to inadequate oxygenation and/or ventilation. The student shows knowledge of how to rapidly check each potential cause and take immediate corrective action. In addition, the student displays awareness of how to anticipate adverse respiratory effects commonly associated with various anesthetic-related and analgesic agents, quickly recognize them, and respond appropriately. For example, the student shows awareness that propofol administration is associated with risk of apnea, particularly with too rapid administration. If this were to occur, the student demonstrates knowledge of how to administer positive pressure ventilations with oxygen until the animal resumes spontaneous respiration. In addition, the student displays knowledge of how to recognize hypoventilation and take appropriate remedial steps, such as reducing the vaporizer setting to the minimum anesthetic depth needed to perform the procedure, correctly administering positive-pressure ventilations (assisting or controlling ventilation), and addressing the cause of hypoventilation, when possible, while alerting the veterinarian.

- The student demonstrates knowledge of how to rapidly recognize and respond to cardiovascular complications, such as cardiac dysrhythmias. The student shows appreciation of the importance of being proactive by anticipating adverse cardiovascular effects commonly associated with various anesthetic-related and analgesic agents; quickly recognizing them; and responding appropriately. For example, if an alpha$_2$-adrenoreceptor agonist is administered, the student shows awareness of bradycardia as a common adverse effect and demonstrates awareness of the need to have the correct reversal agent prepared and ready to administer on the veterinarian's order.

- The student displays awareness of hypotension as a common anesthetic complication and shows understanding of how to recognize clinically significant blood pressure abnormalities. The student demonstrates knowledge of compensatory responses that may occur in response to hypotension, including increased heart rate and vasomotor tone, leading to abnormalities in mucous membrane color, capillary refill time, urine output, and/or body temperature. The student demonstrates awareness of the need to have appropriate IV fluids (and/or blood products) and pressor and/or positive inotropic agents prepared and ready to administer on the veterinarian's order. The student demonstrates knowledge of how to calculate fluid boluses correctly and accurately sets the volume to be infused and the administration rate of the bolus on the fluid pump. The student shows understanding of how to carefully monitor fluid administration rates and shows familiarity with signs of overhydration.

- The student shows awareness of the need to closely monitor body temperature during the peri-anesthetic period. The student displays knowledge of common causes of hypothermia and how to take appropriate preventative steps, particularly in neonate and pediatric patients. If hypothermia does occur, the student shows knowledge of how to recognize it and take appropriate therapeutic measures, including use of IV fluids warmed to body temperature, Bair huggers®, Hot Dog® warming systems, circulating warm-water blankets, and other warming devices. The student shows awareness of common causes of hyperthermia during the peri-anesthetic period (including malignant hyperthermia) and displays knowledge of how to take appropriate therapeutic measures, including use of fans, tepid water baths and enemas, and so on.

- The student demonstrates knowledge of how to promptly recognize neuromuscular indicators of excessive CNS depression – for example, profound muscle relaxation, weak pupillary light reflexes, and centered, dilated pupils.

9) **The student demonstrates knowledge of how to respond appropriately to anesthetic emergencies, including correctly administering reversal agents and emergency drugs, as ordered by the veterinarian, and effectively performing suitable resuscitation procedures.**

- The student shows awareness of how to promptly recognize potentially life-threatening anesthetic complications, including signs of respiratory arrest and cardiopulmonary arrest. The student demonstrates recognition of the need to immediately inform the supervisor/ veterinarian.

- The student demonstrates appreciation of the need to make certain that anesthetic reversal agents, emergency drugs and equipment, and crash cart are prepared and readily available in advance of the procedure.
- The student displays the ability to accurately calculate doses and administer appropriate emergency drugs and/or anesthetic reversal agents correctly (i.e., specific antagonists).
- The student demonstrates awareness that emergency drug doses for each patient should be calculated prior to anesthetic induction.
- The student shows knowledge of how to secure a patent airway and correctly administer positive-pressure ventilations with oxygen by anesthetic machine or resuscitation bag (Ambu® bag). The student demonstrates knowledge of how to properly perform cardiopulmonary resuscitation (CPR), according to current standards.

10) **The student properly completes a controlled substance log utilizing either an official controlled substance log or a mock controlled substance log.**

- The student displays knowledge of how to identify a controlled drug based on the FDA-approved label.
- The student shows awareness of the importance of ensuring that the on-hand inventory of a controlled drug must match the running balance in the controlled substance log. The student displays understanding that any discrepancies must immediately be reported to a supervisor.
- The student demonstrates understanding that controlled drug logs must be bound books with nonperforated pages, that logs for schedule II drugs must be

kept separate from the logs of schedule III–V drugs, and that controlled substance logs must be readily retrievable and kept for a minimum of two years. The student shows awareness that state regulations may require that the logs be kept for a longer period of time.

- The student demonstrates the ability to properly complete a controlled substance log according to applicable federal and state regulations.

11) **The student demonstrates the ability to accurately record and properly maintain anesthesia records.**

- The student demonstrates understanding of the importance of maintaining an anesthetic record for each patient, both as legal documentation of significant events and to facilitate identification of trends in monitored values, thereby allowing early recognition of potential complications.
- The student correctly records relevant information regarding the patient, anesthetic protocol, and procedure in a timely manner. This includes, but is not limited to, the patient's name, body weight, baseline vital signs (including pain score), the procedure to be performed, drug names and doses, times and routes of administration of drugs given, ET tube size, type of breathing circuit, and times of intubation and extubation. The student initializes all entries as appropriate.
- The student properly corrects errors in the record by putting a single line through the mistaken entry and initializing. If using an electronic medical record, the student properly corrects an error by entering an addendum that includes time, date, corrected information, and initials.
- The student accurately records cardiovascular, respiratory, and CNS parameters a minimum of every five minutes in the anesthesia log.

- The student accurately records the percent of gas anesthetic, fresh gas flow rate, and IV fluid rate a minimum of every five minutes.
- The student accurately records treatments of any anesthetic complications that may have occurred. This includes, but is not limited to, the administration of an IV fluid bolus, the administration of an additional analgesic, anesthetic or reversal agent, the administration of a pressor agent, or a change in the rate of a constant rate infusion.
- The student accurately records the start and end times of the anesthesia as well as the procedure. The student clearly identifies when a second procedure begins and ends if appropriate.
- The student demonstrates the ability to accurately interpret anesthesia logs to ensure that the logs are properly recorded and maintained.

4.2 Management and Use of Anesthetic Equipment

12) **The student properly operates and cares for anesthetic equipment and monitoring instruments, demonstrating the ability to detect and appropriately address equipment malfunction or failure.**
    - Given the requirements of the anesthetic protocol and individual patient, the student selects the appropriate anesthetic machine, breathing circuit, reservoir bag, and monitoring instruments.
    - In advance of the procedure, the student completes a pre-anesthetic checklist of all anesthetic delivery and monitoring instruments to make certain that all equipment is in proper working order and free of leaks.
    - The student displays knowledge of the parts of an anesthetic machine, how it delivers anesthetic agents, how it

removes waste gases, and how gas flows through the system.
    - The student demonstrates the ability to correctly operate and adjust the anesthetic machine and monitoring equipment.
    - The student can recognize and respond appropriately to equipment malfunctions or improper equipment setup.
    - The student demonstrates understanding of the importance of checking the patient when equipment malfunctions or improper setup is suspected.

13) **The student demonstrates understanding of the clinical significance of pulse oximetry and correctly operates and cares for pulse oximeters.**
    - The student demonstrates understanding of normal gas exchange and the pertinent respiratory anatomy and physiology as they relate to oxygenation. In addition, the student displays understanding of the oxyhemoglobin dissociation curve to appropriately assess the patient's oxygenation based on the pulse oximetry reading.
    - The student demonstrates understanding of how the pulse oximeter obtains oxygen saturation readings.
    - The student correctly sets up and operates the pulse oximeter, properly placing the probe in an appropriate location based on the patient and procedure.
    - The student shows understanding that accurate pulse oximeter readings are dependent on placing the probe on a well-perfused nonpigmented area.
    - The student demonstrates understanding that pulse oximetry may be used to assess adequacy of oxygenation because pulse oximetry measures arterial hemoglobin saturation with oxygen as SpO_2 or SaO_2.
    - The student shows knowledge of acceptable SpO_2 or SaO_2 levels, and correctly differentiates them from hypoxemia.
    - The student displays awareness of the causes of inaccurate readings, such as

higher oxygen flow rates (Thomas and Lerche, 2024).

21) **The student demonstrates knowledge of, correctly uses, sets up, and cares for sources of oxygen and other gases.**

- The student demonstrates functional knowledge of oxygen and other gas sources, including gas cylinders, oxygen concentrators, and gas lines. For common oxygen tank sizes, including E, H, and T tanks, the student demonstrates knowledge of the relationship between pressure and content. The student displays understanding of the functions of pressure gauges and reads them correctly.

- The student displays knowledge of the functions of and correct settings for pressure regulators (pressure-reducing valves).

- The student properly identifies gas cylinders, gas lines, and outlets by color coding. The student demonstrates understanding of the cylinder yoke and pin-indexed safety system.

- The student correctly attaches gas cylinders and gas lines to the anesthetic machine.

- The student regularly checks pressure gauges to ensure adequate gas remains in tanks. The student is alert to abnormal readings on pressure gauges and responds appropriately.

- The student demonstrates knowledge of the functions of O_2 flowmeters and operates them correctly.

- The student properly stores gas cylinders so that they are attached to yokes, secured to specifically designed carts, or chained to a wall, making certain they are kept in cool, dry areas. The student regularly checks cylinders and gas lines for defects.

22) **The student correctly operates and cares for blood pressure monitors.**

- The student accurately defines the terms *systolic pressure, diastolic pressure,* and *mean arterial pressure.* The student displays understanding of the clinical significance of those terms.

- The student shows awareness that direct monitors provide more accurate measurement of blood pressure than indirect monitors.

- The student displays knowledge of indirect blood pressure monitors, including oscillometric and Doppler devices. The student shows understanding of how these monitors measure blood pressure. The student shows awareness of inaccuracies associated with each type of monitor in smaller patients.

- The student displays knowledge that the Doppler measurement approximates the systolic pressure in dogs but underestimates the systolic pressure in cats by 15 mmHg (Thomas and Lerche, 2024).

- The student correctly uses blood pressure monitoring devices to attain reasonably accurate measures of arterial blood pressure. The student selects a cuff of appropriate width; while the acceptable range for cuff width is 30–50% of the limb circumference, a cuff that is 40% of limb circumference is ideal. The student properly places the cuff around an appendage or the tail. For the Doppler method, the student properly clips fur over the artery, places gel on the probe, and places the probe over the artery, distal to the cuff, ensuring that there is an audible pulse (Thomas and Lerche, 2024).

- The student shows understanding that a cuff that fits too loosely will give falsely high readings and a cuff that fits too tightly will cause the distension of veins. The student also displays understanding that a cuff that is too wide will result in readings that are falsely low and a cuff that is too narrow will result in readings that are falsely high (Thomas and Lerche, 2024).

- The student demonstrates knowledge of acceptable values for arterial blood pressure. In addition, the student demonstrates understanding of values for arterial blood pressure that may indicate hypertension and hypotension.

- The student correctly cares for and cleans blood pressure monitoring devices, following the manufacturer's recommendations.

23) **The student correctly uses and cares for laryngoscopes.**

- The student properly uses the laryngoscope, choosing a suitable blade for the size and species of animal and correctly positioning the blade.
- The student shows awareness that the use of a laryngoscope is recommended for all intubations, even when intubation can be accomplished without it, because laryngoscope use allows oropharyngeal examination and reduces the risk of traumatic intubation by allowing clearer visualization of anatomical structures (Mosley, 2015).
- The student makes certain the laryngoscope blade has been cleaned and disinfected/sterilized prior to use, according to the manufacturer's recommendations.
- The student properly cares for and maintains the laryngoscope and blades

according to the manufacturer's recommendations. The student makes certain the laryngoscope is kept ready for use when needed, with batteries charged and the lamp or fiberoptic light pipe replaced as needed.

24) **The student correctly uses and cares for temperature monitoring devices (e.g., thermometer, etc.).**

- The student correctly uses a variety of temperature monitoring devices, such as digital thermometers and esophageal or rectal temperature probes.
- The student uses protective thermometer covers when taking a rectal temperature to reduce the risk of disease transmission (McCommon, 2022).
- When taking rectal temperature, the student applies appropriate lubricant and gently inserts the thermometer into the rectum in a manner that avoids tissue trauma.
- The student makes certain that the thermometer probe cover is removed with the thermometer.
- The student makes certain that temperature monitoring devices are appropriately cleaned/disinfected after each use.

References

American College of Veterinary Anesthesiologists (2009). *ACVA Monitoring Guidelines Update* Retrieved October 4, 2023, from the American College of Veterinary Anesthesia and Analgesia. www.acvaa.org

Brodbelt, D. C., Flaherty, D., and Pettifer, G. R. (2015). Anesthetic risk and informed consent. In *Veterinary Anesthesia and Analgesia: The Fifth Edition of Lumb and Jones* (ed. K. A. Grimm, L. A. Lamont, W. J. Tranquilli, S. A. Greene, and S. A. Robertson), 11–22. Ames: John Wiley & Sons, Inc.

Buell, L. J. (1999). *Postoperative Opioid Analgesia in Dogs and Cats: An Analysis of the Pharmacological and Clinical Effects of Strong Agonists Relative to Mixed Agonist-Antagonists* [Master's thesis]. Valhalla: New York Medical College.

Buell, L. J. and Schenkel, L. E. (2017). Anesthesia. In *Assessing Essential Skills of Veterinary Technology Students* (ed. L. J. Buell, L. E. Schenkel, and S. Timperman), 25–35. Ames: John Wiley & Sons, Inc.

Cambridge, A., Tobias, K., and Newberry, R. (2000). Subjective and objective measurement of postoperative pain in cats. *J Am Vet Med Assoc* 217(5): 685–690.

Fox, S., and Mellor, D. L. (1998). Changes in plasma cortisol concentrations in bitches in response to different combinations of halothane and butorphanol, with or without ovariohysterectomy. *Res Vet Sci*: 125–133.

Hansen, B., and Hardie, E. (1993). Prescription and use of analgesics in dogs and cats in a veterinary teaching hospital: 258 cases. *J Am Vet Med Assoc* 202(9): 1485–1494.

Hardie, E. M., Hansen, B. D., and Carroll, G. S. (1997). Behavior after ovariohysterectomy in the dog: what's normal? *Appl Anim Behav Sci* 51: 111–128.

Hellyer, P. W., and Gaynor, J. S. (1998). Acute postsurgical pain in dogs and cats. *Compen Contin Educ Prac Vet*, 20(2), 140–153.

Holton, L. L., Scott, E. M., Nolan, A. M., Reid, J., and Welsh, E. (1998). Relationship between physiological factors and clinical pain in dogs scored using a numerical rating scale. *J Small Anim Pract* 39(10): 469–474.

McCommon, G. W. (2022). History and physical examination. In *McCurnin's Clinical Textbook for Veterinary Technicians*, 10th e (ed. J. M. Bassert, and J. A. Thomas), 217–218. St. Louis: Elsevier.

Mosley, C. A. (2015). Anesthesia. In *Veterinary Anesthesia and Analgesia: The Fifth Edition of Lumb and Jones* (ed. K. A. Grimm, L. A. Lamont, W. J. Tranquilli, S. A. Greene, and S. A. Robertson), 23–85. Ames: John Wiley & Sons, Inc.

Muir III, W. W. (2015). Pain and stress. In *Handbook of Veterinary Pain Management,* 3rd e (ed. J. S. Gaynor and W. W. Muir III, 42–60. St. Louis: Elsevier.

Quandt, J. E., Lee, J. A., and Powell, L. L. (2005). Analgesia in critically ill patients. *Compen Contin Educ Prac Vet* 27(6): 433–445.

Tear, M. (2022). *Small Animal Surgical Nursing* (4th ed.) (p. 19). St. Louis: Elsevier.

Thomas, J. A., and Lerche, P. (2024). *Anesthesia and Analgesia for Veterinary Technicians*, 6th e. (pp. 106, 138, 140–141, 143, 216–217, 229). St. Louis: Elsevier.

Veterinary Anesthesia and Analgesia Support Group (2011). *Anesthetic Induction Routine* Retrieved from Veterinary Anesthesia and Analgesia Support Group. www.vasg.org/anesthetic_induction.htm.

Wiese, A. J. (2015). Assessing pain. In *Handbook of Veterinary Pain Management* (ed. J. S. Gaynor and W. W. Muir III, W. W., 3rd e). 67–97. St. Louis: Elsevier.

Wiese, A. J., Muir III, W. W., and Wittum, T. E. (2005). Characteristics of pain and response to analgesic treatment in dogs and cats examined at a veterinary teaching hospital emergency service. *J Amer Vet Med Assoc* 226(12): 2004–2009.

Wiese, A. J., and Yaksh, T. L. (2015). Nociception and pain mechanisms. In *Handbook of Veterinary Pain Management* (ed. J. S. Gaynor and W. W. Muir III, W. W., 3rd e). 10–41. St. Louis: Elsevier.

5

Surgical Nursing and Assisting

Sandra Lynn Bertholf, MS, LVT and Lisa E. Schenkel, DVM, CCRT, CVMA

5.1 Fundamentals of Common Surgical Procedures

1) **The student displays knowledge of ovariohysterectomy in dogs and cats.**
   - The student demonstrates knowledge of the pertinent anatomy and physiology.
   - The student correctly explains ovariohysterectomy as the surgical removal of the uterus and ovaries.
   - The student demonstrates knowledge of correct patient preparation and positioning, anesthesia and analgesia, surgical assisting, aftercare, and necessary equipment and instrumentation for ovariohysterectomy in dogs and cats.
   - The student displays understanding of the effects of ovariohysterectomy on the health and behavior of dogs and cats.
   - The student shows awareness of considerations regarding age and the estrous cycle in scheduling ovariohysterectomy in dogs and cats.
   - The student displays knowledge of common complications associated with ovariohysterectomy in dogs and cats.
2) **The student demonstrates knowledge of Cesarean section.**
   - The student demonstrates knowledge of the pertinent anatomy and physiology.
   - The student correctly explains Cesarean section as removal of the fetus through an incision in the abdominal wall and uterus. Student demonstrates knowledge that Cesarean section is a surgical procedure for dystocia or medical emergency during pregnancy, such as pelvic fracture.
   - The student shows awareness of the breeds, as well as the predisposing anatomic factors, that are expected to require Caesarean section, for example, the English Bulldog.
   - The student demonstrates knowledge of correct patient preparation and positioning, anesthesia and analgesia, surgical assisting, aftercare, and necessary equipment and instrumentation for Cesarean section.
   - The student demonstrates awareness of common complications associated with Cesarean section.
   - The student displays knowledge of how to properly prepare an appropriate environment for the newborns (i.e., a clean, dry area with plenty of towels).
   - The student correctly explains appropriate steps to take to initiate spontaneous respiration and achieve cardiovascular stability in the newborn. The student describes the proper procedure for

Assessing Essential Skills of Veterinary Technology Students, Fourth Edition. Edited by Lisa E. Schenkel, Amanda Colón, Sandra Lynn Bertholf, Sabrina Timperman, and Laurie J. Buell.
© 2024 John Wiley & Sons, Inc. Published 2024 by John Wiley & Sons, Inc.
Companion website: www.wiley.com/go/Schenkel/AssessingEssentialSkillsofVeterinaryTechnologyStudents4e

ligating the umbilicus and reuniting the newborn with the mother.

3) **The student displays knowledge of orthopedic procedures.**
- The student demonstrates knowledge of the pertinent anatomy and physiology.
- The student displays awareness of orthopedic procedures as those involving the skeleton, joints, and associated structures.
- The student shows understanding of orthopedic terms and abbreviations, such as cranial cruciate ligament (CCL), medial patellar luxation (MPL), and intervertebral disk disease (IVDD).
- The student demonstrates knowledge of correct patient preparation and positioning, anesthesia and analgesia, surgical assisting, aftercare, and necessary equipment and instrumentation for orthopedic procedures.
- The student displays awareness of the benefits of rehabilitation therapy as part of the post-operative care of the orthopedic patient.

4) **The student displays knowledge of orchiectomy in common species.**
- The student demonstrates knowledge of the pertinent anatomy and physiology.
- The student displays awareness of castration as removal of the testes.
- The student demonstrates knowledge of correct patient preparation and positioning, anesthesia and analgesia, surgical assisting, aftercare, and necessary equipment and instrumentation for orchiectomy.
- The student displays knowledge of the effects of orchiectomy on the health and behavior of dogs and cats.
- The student shows awareness of considerations regarding age on the scheduling of orchiectomy in dogs and cats.
- The student shows awareness of common complications associated with orchiectomy.

5) **The student displays knowledge of tail docking.**
- The student demonstrates knowledge of the pertinent anatomy.

- The student demonstrates understanding that the term *tail docking* generally refers to the partial amputation of the tail for aesthetic reasons; however, tail amputation may be medically necessary to treat trauma, infection, or neoplasia of the tail.
- The student demonstrates knowledge of correct patient preparation and positioning, anesthesia and analgesia, surgical assisting, aftercare, and necessary equipment and instrumentation for tail docking.
- The student displays awareness of the common complications associated with tail docking and tail amputation.

6) **The student displays knowledge of onychectomy in dogs and cats.**
- The student demonstrates knowledge of the pertinent anatomy.
- The student demonstrates awareness of onychectomy in cats as surgical amputation of the distal phalanx (P3) and claw, and in dogs as surgical removal of the dewclaw.
- The student demonstrates knowledge of correct patient preparation and positioning, anesthesia and analgesia, surgical assisting, aftercare, and necessary equipment and instrumentation for onychectomy.
- The student displays awareness of common complications associated with onychectomy.
- The student shows awareness of considerations regarding age on the scheduling of onychectomy in cats.
- The student demonstrates awareness that onychectomy for any reason other than when it is medically necessary is illegal in certain states or cities.

7) **The student displays knowledge of laparotomy.**
- The student demonstrates knowledge of the pertinent anatomy and physiology.
- The student demonstrates knowledge of general indications for laparotomy in all common species, for example, the presence of abdominal foreign bodies,

trauma, gastric dilatation volvulus, or abdominal masses.

- The student displays awareness that laparotomy is a surgical incision through the abdominal wall.
- The student demonstrates knowledge of correct patient preparation and positioning, anesthesia and analgesia, surgical assisting, aftercare, and necessary equipment and instrumentation for laparotomy.
- The student displays awareness of the common complications associated with laparotomy as well as complications related to specific indications.

8) **The student displays knowledge of dystocia in common species.**
   - The student demonstrates knowledge of the pertinent anatomy and physiology.
   - The student demonstrates awareness that dystocia is a difficult birth.
   - The student shows knowledge that dystocia is more prevalent in certain breeds, for example, chondrodystrophic breeds.
   - The student displays knowledge of normal stages of labor as well as the criteria for dystocia.
   - The student shows awareness that dystocia is an emergency situation requiring prompt veterinary intervention.
   - The student displays knowledge of potential complications of dystocia.

9) **The student displays knowledge of dehorning in cattle and goats.**
   - The student demonstrates knowledge of the pertinent anatomy.
   - The student displays knowledge that dehorning is the removal of the horns.
   - The student explains the overall benefit of dehorning in the management of ruminants.
   - The student displays knowledge of different dehorning techniques and equipment used in animals of different ages as well as different ruminant species. For example, it is recommended that cattle be dehorned at the age of two to three months, which is before the horn is firmly attached to the skull. In small ruminants, it is recommended that dehorning take place before the age of two to three weeks when the procedure will be less painful and less likely to cause an infection. Although a Barnes dehorner can be used in cattle, it is not recommended in goats due to the risk of skull fracture (Samples et al., 2022). The student demonstrates knowledge of correct patient preparation and positioning, anesthesia and analgesia, surgical assisting, aftercare, and necessary equipment and instrumentation for dehorning in cattle and goats.
   - The student displays recognition that the use of a multimodal approach to analgesia, including the use of a local anesthetic, an anti-inflammatory agent, and, when possible, a sedative-analgesic agent, is recommended to diminish the acute phase of pain associated with dehorning (Stock, Baldridge, Griffin et al., 2013).
   - The student displays knowledge of potential complications of dehorning. For example, the student demonstrates knowledge that once the horns are attached to the skull, dehorning becomes more difficult and results in exposure of the frontal sinus, which may take up to six weeks to close (Samples et al., 2022).

10) **The student displays knowledge of the correction of prolapsed organs.**
   - The student demonstrates knowledge of the pertinent anatomy and physiology.
   - The student demonstrates awareness of organ prolapse as displacement of that organ. For example, uterine prolapse occurs when the uterus becomes everted so that the cervix is displaced through the vaginal orifice.
   - The student displays knowledge of common types of organ prolapse, in which species they occur, and how frequently they occur. For example, prolapse of the nictitans gland is the most common disorder affecting the third eyelid in dogs.

- The student demonstrates awareness of the types of organ prolapse that are emergency situations requiring prompt veterinary intervention.
- The student demonstrates knowledge of correct patient preparation and positioning, anesthesia and analgesia, surgical assisting, aftercare, and necessary equipment and instrumentation for correction of various types of organ prolapse.
- The student displays knowledge of potential complications of common types of prolapsed organs.

5.2 Experience with Common Surgical Procedures

11) **The student takes an appropriate active role in the ovariohysterectomy of a dog and a cat.**
    - The student displays understanding of the procedure and the relevant anatomy.
    - The student properly prepares all equipment and instrumentation prior to anesthetic induction. The student accurately calculates doses of prescribed anesthetic and analgesic agents.
    - The student properly draws up and administers prescribed anesthetics and analgesics.
    - The student correctly assists in the procedure, as directed by the veterinarian.
    - The student provides appropriate aftercare for the patient.
12) **The student takes an appropriate active role in the orchiectomy of a dog and a cat.**
    - The student displays understanding of the procedure and the relevant anatomy.
    - The student properly prepares all equipment and instrumentation prior to anesthetic induction. The student accurately calculates doses of prescribed anesthetic and analgesic agents.

- The student properly draws up and administers prescribed anesthetics and analgesics.
- The student correctly assists in the procedure, as directed by the veterinarian.
- The student provides appropriate aftercare for the patient.

5.3 Management of the Veterinary Surgical Patient

13) **The student displays awareness of the need to confirm patient identities, making certain that they correctly match scheduled surgical procedures.**
    - The student shows appreciation of the need for diligence in the use of medical records, signalment, and animal identification methods to make certain that the patient and scheduled surgical procedure correctly match. For example, the patient's name and signalment must be matched to its medical record upon admission to the facility and before every treatment. In addition, the patient's medical problem(s) and reason for surgery must be confirmed. The student displays recognition of the importance of properly labeling the patient's cage with all pertinent information.
    - In facilities using ID bands, the student shows awareness that the band must be attached before the animal is taken from the owner and rechecked prior to every procedure and/or treatment.
14) **The student demonstrates understanding of the need to make certain medical records are in order and all necessary consent forms are properly completed and signed prior to patients undergoing surgical procedures.**
    - The student displays the ability to correctly organize and make appropriate, legible entries in medical records, using correct spelling, abbreviations, and format.

- The student demonstrates appreciation of medical records and consent forms as legal documents and displays understanding of how to treat them as such.

15) **The student demonstrates the ability to carefully and knowledgeably review pre-operative assessment.**
    - Prior to and during the pre-anesthetic period, the student displays awareness of how to appropriately work with the veterinarian to gather as much information as possible on the patient relevant to anesthesia, analgesia, and the procedure.
    - The student shows understanding of the need to review the patient's medical records to make certain all pre-procedural tests ordered by the veterinarian have been completed. The student demonstrates awareness that minimum laboratory evaluation includes complete blood count (CBC), blood chemistries, and urinalysis and displays understanding of why each test is necessary. The student displays knowledge of additional diagnostic tests that the veterinarian may order prior to the procedure and the purposes of each, including, but not limited to, ECG, coagulation tests, and/or radiographs.
    - The student demonstrates the ability to understand the results of pre-operative evaluation and explain their pertinence to anesthesia, analgesia, and the procedure.

16) **The student demonstrates the ability to correctly assess up-to-the-minute patient status during the peri-anesthetic period.**
    - The student demonstrates understanding of how to correctly conduct a brief physical examination prior to the procedure, not to replicate veterinarian's prior physical examination, but to obtain vital signs, help determine baseline parameters in the awake animal (which later can be compared with those obtained during and after anesthesia), and aid in

the discovery of any acute abnormalities in the period immediately preceding anesthetic induction.

- The student displays knowledge of how to carefully observe the behavior of the patient prior to the procedure. This is to help detect any behaviors associated with pain and is equally important in animals not thought to be experiencing pain, because it allows comparison with the patient's behavior after the procedure. The student shows awareness that deviation from the individual animal's normal behaviors may be evidence of pain (e.g., inability to sleep, anorexia, depression, apprehensiveness, normally friendly animal behaving aggressively or unwilling to interact, lack of grooming in cats, etc.) (Wiese, 2015).
- The student displays understanding of how to distinguish physical or behavioral abnormalities and to effectively and accurately communicate them to the veterinarian.

17) **The student demonstrates the ability to implement an anesthetic protocol in an organized, well-integrated manner.**
    - The student displays the ability to work with the veterinarian to plan and coordinate anesthesia, follow the anesthetic plan in a careful, organized manner, and anticipate and be prepared to respond appropriately to the surgeon's and individual patient's needs.
    - The student demonstrates awareness that the longer the animal is kept under anesthesia, the greater the risk of complications. In coordinating anesthesia, therefore, the student shows knowledge of how to take all possible steps to minimize time under anesthesia. For example, all equipment and drugs necessary for anesthetic induction, maintenance, and recovery should be checked and prepared well in advance of anesthetic induction.

18) **The student correctly locates and safely palpates the urinary bladder. The student carefully expresses the bladder when appropriate and directed by the veterinarian.**

   - The student displays awareness of the importance of allowing an animal to urinate prior to the procedure – for example, to alleviate discomfort and to avoid interference of a distended bladder with the procedure.
   - The student gives the animal adequate opportunity to urinate at an appropriate time prior to anesthetic induction – for example, walking a dog or giving a cat a litter box.
   - The student displays knowledge of the anatomy of the urinary tract and where the bladder is generally located in the individual patient.
   - The student uses correct technique in locating and safely palpating the bladder.
   - The student displays knowledge of risks associated with manual expression of the bladder. For example, even correct manual expression technique can result in hematuria and bladder rupture.
   - The student demonstrates knowledge of conditions in which manual bladder expression would be contraindicated, such as abdominal trauma, urethral obstruction, and cystotomy.
   - When appropriate and directed by the veterinarian, the student uses correct technique in safely and carefully expressing the bladder manually.

19) **The student uses correct aseptic technique to prepare the skin at the surgical site.**

   - The student demonstrates understanding of the need to minimize microbial flora on the skin at the anticipated surgical site in order to decrease the chance of surgical wound contamination.
   - The student demonstrates understanding of appropriate uses and relative advantages and disadvantages of different surgical scrubs and topical antiseptic solutions, such as povidone-iodine, chlorhexidine, and 70% isopropyl alcohol.
   - The student uses the appropriate clipper blade to complete fur clipping for surgical site preparation. The student properly maintains the clipper and blades, including cleaning and disinfecting the clipper and blades between patients, and takes care to avoid skin abrasion or clipper burn.
   - The student demonstrates understanding that fur removal and preliminary skin scrubbing are performed in the prep area. After properly identifying the approximate incision site, the student cleanly and evenly removes the fur, leaving sufficient margins around the anticipated incision site, and thoroughly vacuums loose fur. While the patient is still in the prep area, the student correctly performs the initial skin cleansing with surgical scrub solution to remove gross contamination, wearing exam gloves and mask. The student carefully moves the patient to the surgical suite, properly connecting the patient to the anesthetic machine and monitoring devices and positioning the patient appropriately for the procedure. The student performs the final skin scrub, using correct aseptic technique.

20) **The student demonstrates knowledge of standard positions and properly positions patients for routine surgical procedures.**

   - When appropriate, the student asks the surgeon for any personal preferences in patient positioning.
   - The student positions and secures patients properly in a manner that provides optimal convenience for the surgeon and safety for the patient. The student uses positioning devices appropriately.
   - The student makes certain to keep the airway patent at all times and to connect monitoring devices to the patient in a way that does not interfere with patient

positioning or have the potential to compromise the sterile field.

- The student properly disconnects the endotracheal tube from the breathing circuit prior to positioning the patient and makes certain that the endotracheal tube is properly reconnected to the breathing circuit once the patient has been positioned.
- The student adjusts the surgery table height and lights to meet the needs of the surgeon and procedure.
- The student places appropriate barriers between the patient and surgery table, such as warming devices, towels, and other appropriate barriers.

21) **When providing surgical assistance, the student strictly observes proper operating room conduct and aseptic technique.**

- The student practices proper daily hygiene, including, but not limited to, keeping fingernails clean, smooth, and short, and frequently washing hands. The student demonstrates awareness that the ideal nail length is 2 mm or less to minimize contamination from subungual bacteria (Broaddus, 2018). The student displays awareness that nail polish is not recommended, hair should be pulled back, and jewelry should be removed prior to entering the surgical suite in order to avoid these items inadvertently falling into or otherwise contaminating the surgical field (Bassert, 2022). The student avoids the use of perfume or other scents because they can be objectionable to others when working in close quarters and have the potential to mask the odors of anesthetic gases (Tear, 2022).
- The student shows awareness that any person entering the surgical suite must wash their hands thoroughly and wear a cap, mask, and clean surgical scrubs or a gown. The student makes certain to wear only clean shoes in the operating room and follows facility protocol regarding the use of shoe covers.

- The student correctly distinguishes between sterile and non-sterile personnel. When non-sterile, the student pays constant attention to maintaining aseptic technique and displays appropriate operating room conduct, including, but not limited to, keeping movement and talking to a minimum; not reaching across or over a sterile field; not moving objects unnecessarily in the suite once surgery begins; moving behind (never in front of) sterile personnel; never passing between two sterile surfaces or objects; keeping the door to the surgical suite closed; and monitoring patients and equipment without interfering with the surgeon or team.
- The student demonstrates the ability to correctly scrub in and join the sterile surgical team by: donning a mask, cap and shoe covers; performing a sterile scrub; donning a surgical gown; and performing closed and open gloving.
- When scrubbing in, the student correctly scrubs hands and forearms and dons gowns, gloves, and other sterile attire properly. The student maintains aseptic technique at all times.
- When scrubbed in, the student always keeps their hands and arms in front of the body, above the waist and beneath the shoulders, only touches sterile objects, and moves only in ways that prevent self-contamination, including, but not limited to, facing the surgical field at all times and passing other sterile personnel back-to-back.

22) **Using aseptic technique, the student correctly assists with care of exposed tissues and organs.**

- The student handles tissues gently, demonstrating understanding that great care is necessary to minimize trauma and injury.
- The student observes strict aseptic technique at all times when caring for exposed tissues and organs.

- When assisting in retraction, the student carefully and properly positions handheld retractors, making certain they are well stabilized to prevent slippage.
- The student displays awareness that exposed tissues and organs must be kept moist to avoid desiccation. The student shows understanding of why lavage (or irrigation) fluids should be sterile, isotonic, and buffered. The student properly prepares sterile irrigation fluids, warming them when appropriate, and correctly supplies them to surgeon.

23) **The student correctly performs the aseptic surgical scrub and drying of hands.**
    - The student correctly prepares for the aseptic scrub by donning a cap and mask and removing all jewelry prior to starting surgical scrub.
    - The student demonstrates appropriate scrub technique, using either counted brush strokes or the timed method.
    - The student rinses hands/arms with water using aseptic technique.
    - The student dries hands/arms with a sterile towel using aseptic technique.

24) **The student demonstrates aseptic technique when donning a surgical mask, cap, gown, and gloves.**
    - The student correctly dons a cap and mask prior to starting an aseptic surgical scrub of the hands/arms.
    - The student properly dons a sterile gown by correctly identifying the sleeve openings and unfolding the sterile gown without it touching any surfaces that are not sterile. The student correctly utilizes a non-sterile assistant to tie the gown around the neck and waist of the student.
    - The student appropriately dons surgical gloves using aseptic technique after donning a cap/mask/gown and completing an aseptic scrub of the hands/arms.

- The student demonstrates awareness of the sterile area of a gown and maintains correct operating room conduct to maintain sterility while gowned.

25) **The student properly passes instruments and supplies.**
    - The student correctly identifies common surgical instruments, knows the appropriate terminology for each, and demonstrates knowledge of their proper uses.
    - The student correctly distinguishes sterile instruments and supplies from those that are non-sterile.
    - The student properly passes sterile items to sterile personnel, maintaining strict aseptic technique.

26) **The student displays knowledge of how to correctly operate and care for suction and cautery devices.**
    - The student demonstrates understanding of how to properly set up both suction and cautery devices, checking that they are functioning properly in advance of the procedure.
    - The student shows awareness of how to correctly prepare necessary attachments and parts in advance, anticipating the surgeon's needs.
    - The student demonstrates familiarity with how to operate suction and cautery devices.
    - The student displays knowledge of the proper cleaning, disinfection and/or sterilization of the various parts of suction and cautery devices.
    - The student shows awareness of safety concerns associated with the use of cautery and suction devices, as well as steps necessary to minimize risks.

27) **The student demonstrates knowledge of principles of operation and proper care of fiberoptic equipment.**
    - The student demonstrates familiarity with the difference between flexible and rigid scopes. The student shows awareness that flexible scopes generally are

37) **The student correctly prepares gowns, masks, gloves, and drapes.**

- The student displays familiarity with different types of gowns and gown materials, types of masks, gloves, head covers, and protective footwear.
- The student lays out appropriate types and sizes of surgical gloves for the surgical team. The student displays the ability to assist the surgeon in gowning.
- If reusable gowns and drapes are used, the student correctly washes, dries, and folds gowns and drapes after use. The student correctly assembles packs containing gowns or drapes, folding them properly, using appropriate wrap materials, enclosing dependable sterilization indicators, taping them closed, and labeling them properly.
- The student correctly differentiates closed gloving from open gloving and displays the ability to assist the surgeon in changing gloves during procedure.

38) **The student safely operates and properly cares for autoclaves.**

- The student displays awareness of different sizes and types of autoclaves.
- The student correctly identifies instruments and equipment that can be safely sterilized via the autoclaving process.
- The student demonstrates understanding of the autoclaving process and how it produces sterilization, when functioning properly.
- The student correctly and safely operates the autoclave according to the manufacturer's recommendations, filling it with distilled water to the appropriate level, determining the proper time, temperature, and pressure requirements to sterilize each instrument and/or pack, and properly loading it for optimal performance.
- The student displays familiarity with various types of packaging material and selects the appropriate type for each item.

- The student properly determines when the autoclaving cycle is complete and vents the autoclave at the correct time.
- The student safely removes items from the autoclave.
- The student displays knowledge of the various types of sterilization indicators and the proper use of each.
- The student stores sterilized instruments, packs, and supplies appropriately.

39) **The student correctly differentiates disinfection from sterilization and properly utilizes various methods of disinfection and sterilization.**

- The student displays awareness that sterilization destroys all microorganisms and pathogenic matter on inanimate objects, while disinfection destroys or inhibits growth of most microorganisms and pathogenic matter on inanimate objects.
- The student shows understanding that cold sterilization involves immersion of an object in a disinfectant solution and may be used to achieve different levels of disinfection, depending on the concentration used and the contact time (Reuss-Lamky, 2017).
- The student properly utilizes agents such as glutaraldehyde and benzalkonium chloride solutions for cold sterilization. The student wears gloves when preparing or touching cold sterilization solutions.
- The student safely and properly utilizes various sterilization methods, including autoclaving and gas sterilization (e.g., ethylene oxide and/or gas plasma). The student displays knowledge of potential hazards associated with ethylene oxide sterilization as well as limitations of gas sterilization methods.
- The student demonstrates awareness that cold sterilization is appropriate only in limited circumstances, such as disinfection of instruments or equipment that

would be damaged by other means of sterilization.

- The student demonstrates knowledge of procedures requiring sterilized instruments – for example, those in which an instrument touches tissues under the skin (Reuss-Lamky, 2017).

40) **The student correctly and efficiently sets up all needed instrumentation and equipment prior to the surgical procedure.**

- The student demonstrates knowledge of all instrumentation and equipment necessary for common surgical procedures.
- The student checks all instruments and equipment in advance of the procedure to ensure that it is in proper working order.
- The student handles all instrumentation and equipment properly, maintaining aseptic technique when appropriate.
- The student makes certain that surgical setup is properly completed prior to anesthetic induction to minimize the patient's time under anesthesia.

41) **The student demonstrates knowledge of the correct names and proper uses of commonly used instruments.**

- The student correctly identifies by name specific surgical instruments and groups them into such categories as scalpel blades, scalpel handles, scissors, hemostats, needle holders, towel clamps, forceps, retractors (handheld and self-retaining), orthopedic instruments, etc.
- The student displays understanding of appropriate uses of specific, commonly used instruments. For example, Kelly forceps are hemostats used to crush blood vessels, Metzenbaum scissors are used to cut delicate tissues, Backhaus towel clamps are used to secure drapes to the patient, etc.
- The student displays knowledge of the instruments that are likely to be required for common surgical procedures and which instruments should be included in specific, multi-instrument packs.

42) **The student displays the ability to accurately identify types and sizes of suture materials and needles.**

- The student demonstrates the ability to differentiate between monofilament and braided, absorbable and non-absorbable, and synthetic and natural suture materials.
- The student recognizes both generic and common brand names for suture materials.
- The student displays understanding of conventions for sizing the diameter of suture material, particularly for suture sized below 1. For example, a 2-0 suture has a smaller diameter than a 1-0 suture, and a 1-0 suture has a smaller diameter than 0.
- The student properly distinguishes between swaged needles and eyed needles.
- The student shows knowledge of commonly used types and sizes of suture needles, including, but not limited to, cutting, taper, reverse cutting, etc.
- The student demonstrates familiarity with common uses of various types of suture needles and suture materials.

43) **The student properly cleans and maintains the operating room.**

- The student demonstrates knowledge of effective cleaning protocols and uses detergent/disinfectant solutions appropriate for cleaning specific surfaces or objects. The student displays knowledge of the amount of contact time necessary for each type to achieve effective disinfection.
- The student damp wipes all horizontal surfaces before the first surgery of the day to minimize airborne contaminants. The student cleans the operating room at the end of each procedure, prior to the entry of the next patient (Tear, 2022). At the end of every day, even when the operating room has not been used, the student cleans all surfaces (including the floor) and equipment with

disinfectant solution, taking care to wipe lights (to prevent dust from falling onto the sterile field). The student demonstrates awareness that ideally, the surgery suite should have a separate mop (from the rest of the hospital) or if not available, then the surgery suite floor should be cleaned first (prior to the rest of the hospital).

- The student demonstrates awareness that, at least once a week, all equipment and supplies should be removed from the operating room and all surfaces, including floors, walls, doors, door handles, wheels, foot pedals, lights, and so on, and scrubbed with an appropriate detergent/disinfectant solution. All equipment also should be cleaned with an appropriate detergent/disinfectant solution.
- The student keeps cleaning implements and buckets designated for operating room use only separated from other cleaning equipment. To minimize microbial contamination, the student makes certain that cleaning implements and buckets are thoroughly washed, rinsed, and allowed to dry prior to being stored.

44) **The student displays knowledge of how to properly maintain aseptic technique in the operating room.**
   - The student demonstrates appreciation of the importance of keeping the surgical area as free of microorganisms as possible.
   - The student accurately demarcates the entire sterile field.
   - The student shows understanding of proper operating room conduct. For example, sterile personnel should only touch sterile items and non-sterile personnel should only touch non-sterile items.
   - The student demonstrates knowledge of how to correctly introduce items into a sterile field while maintaining sterility;

for example, how to properly open wraps and pouches, how to appropriately transfer instruments, and how to correctly pour irrigation fluids.
   - The student displays understanding of how to move in a manner that maintains the integrity of the sterile field. The student shows awareness that movement should be minimized to decrease air currents that could contaminate the sterile field.
   - The student shows appreciation of the importance of restricting conversation and keeping the door to the operating room closed as much as possible.
   - The student displays understanding of the importance of immediately reporting and correcting any violation of aseptic technique (Tear, 2022).

45) **The student properly cleans the operating room following surgical procedures.**
   - The student safely removes scalpel blades from handles and properly deposits scalpel blades and needles in appropriate sharps containers.
   - The student correctly disposes of used paper items, such as drapes, gauze sponges, masks, disposable gowns, and so on.
   - The student places all used cloth items, such as towels, drapes, gowns, and so on, into detergent solution to presoak. The student demonstrates knowledge that surgical items should be laundered separately from all other laundry.
   - The student makes certain to confirm with the surgeon which tissues, organs, or other organic material must be kept for laboratory analysis, and handles, labels, stores, and packages them appropriately.
   - The student properly disposes of hazardous medical waste.
   - The student carefully and safely removes instruments and packs from the operating room. The student removes organic material such as blood or tissue from instruments as soon as possible to prevent pitting and/or corrosion, presoaking

them in an appropriate instrument cleaning solution. Making certain that box locks and ratchets are open, the student correctly and thoroughly cleans, rinses, lubricates (when appropriate), and dries instruments. The student checks each instrument to make certain it is in good repair and functioning properly.

- The student makes certain to shut off warming and monitoring devices, gas cylinders and lines, surgical lights, cautery and suction equipment, and scavenging systems.
- The student soaks rebreathing bags, anesthetic hoses, and so on in appropriate disinfectant solution, rinses them thoroughly, and hangs them to dry completely prior to use.
- The student correctly cleans the operating room after each procedure.

References

Bassert, J. M. and Lazo, T. (2022). Introduction to veterinary nursing and technology; its laws and ethics. In; J. M. Bassert, A. D. Beal, O. M. Samples, *McCurnin's Clinical Textbook for Veterinary Technicians and Nurses* (10th ed.) (p. 17). St. Louis: Elsevier.

Broaddus, Kristyn D (2018). Nail polish & bacterial counts in surgery, *Clinicians Brief*. Retrieved June 6, 2023, from https://www.cliniciansbrief.com/article/nail-polish-bacterial-counts-surgery.

Buell, L. J. and Schenkel, L. E. (2017). Surgical nursing and assisting. In *Assessing Essential Skills of Veterinary Technology Students*, 3rd e. (ed. L. J. Buell, L. E. Schenkel, and S. Timperman), 37–47. Ames: John Wiley & Sons, Inc.

Committee on Veterinary Technician Education and Activities (2023). Accreditation Policies and Procedures of the AVMA Committee on Veterinary Technician Education and Activities (CVTEA). Retrieved August 17, 2023, from https://www.avma.org/education/center-for-veterinary-accreditation/committee-veterinary-technician-education-activities.

Lichtenbarger, M. (2005). Gastrointestinal endoscopy: procedures and equipment care. *Vet Tech* 26(6): 404–416.

McCommon, G. W. (2022). Surgical instruments and aseptic technique. In *McCurnin's Clinical Textbook for Veterinary Technicians and Nurses*, 10th e. (ed. J. M. Bassert, A. D. Beal, O. M. Samples), 1001–1006. St. Louis: Elsevier.

Reuss-Lamky, H. (2017). Keys to successful high-level disinfection and sterilization processes. *Today's Veterinary Nurse*. Retrieved June 6, 2023 from https://todaysveterinarynurse.com/infectious-disease/keys-to-successful-high-level-disinfection-and-sterilization-processes/

Samples, O. M., Geeding, A. A., Trenta, M. L. and Vallotton, D. B. (2022). Large animal surgical nursing. In *McCurnin's Clinical Textbook for Veterinary Technicians and Nurses*, 10th e. (ed. J. M. Bassert, A. D. Beal, O. M. Samples), 1105–1106. St. Louis: Elsevier.

Stock, M. L., Baldridge, S. L., Griffin, D., et al. (2013, March). Bovine dehorning: assessing pain and providing analgesic management. *Vet Clin North Am Food Anim Pract* 29(1): 103–133.

Tear, M. (2022). *Small Animal Surgical Nursing Skills and Concepts*, 4th e. (pp. 102, 265, 1006). St. Louis: Elsevier.

Wiese, A. J. (2015). Assessing pain. In *Handbook of Veterinary Pain Management*, 3rd e. (ed. J. S. Gaynor and W. W. Muir III), 67–97. St. Louis: Elsevier.

6

Clinical Laboratory Procedures

Lisa E. Schenkel, DVM, CCRT, CVMA, Amanda Colón, DVM,
and Sandra Lynn Bertholf, MS, LVT

6.1 Management of Laboratory Specimens and Equipment

1) **The student properly chooses and cares for laboratory equipment.**
   - The student describes the functions of common pieces of laboratory equipment. Based on this understanding, the student correctly chooses equipment for the requested test procedure.
   - The student displays awareness of the importance of organizing and storing equipment-use manuals.
   - The student properly cleans common laboratory equipment according to manufacturers' recommendations.
   - The student properly uses, cleans, and stores the microscope, including, but not limited to, making certain not to leave the oil immersion objective in contact with the immersion oil on the slide.
2) **The student participates in employing quality control procedures.**
   - The student shows understanding of the importance of quality control in achieving accurate results.
   - The student displays understanding of the importance of maintenance logs and uses them appropriately.

- The student participates in performing calibration of common laboratory equipment according to manufacturers' recommendations.
- The student demonstrates the ability to differentiate accurate from incorrect results, considering the individual patient as well as specimen submitted.

3) **The student demonstrates understanding of how to take all necessary steps to maximize the safety of patients, clients, and staff when collecting and handling laboratory specimens.**
   - The student demonstrates knowledge of appropriate laboratory conduct and dress.
   - The student displays understanding of how to safely collect laboratory specimens.
   - The student demonstrates knowledge of the locations of safety features of a laboratory, such as Safety Data Sheets (SDS), fire emergency equipment, emergency exits, eye wash stations and showers, emergency exit maps, and so on. The student displays the ability to appropriately utilize laboratory safety features.
   - The student shows awareness of potential safety hazards and carries out laboratory procedures without breaking safety protocols.

Assessing Essential Skills of Veterinary Technology Students, Fourth Edition. Edited by Lisa E. Schenkel,
Amanda Colón, Sandra Lynn Bertholf, Sabrina Timperman, and Laurie J. Buell.
© 2024 John Wiley & Sons, Inc. Published 2024 by John Wiley & Sons, Inc.
Companion website: www.wiley.com/go/Schenkel/AssessingEssentialSkillsofVeterinaryTechnologyStudents4e

- The student describes the appropriate use of personal protective equipment in the laboratory as well as the proper donning and doffing of personal protective equipment.
- The student displays appreciation of the importance of rigorous hygiene, thoroughly washing hands, wearing gloves when appropriate, and cleaning all work areas with suitable disinfectants after use.
- The student makes certain that no food or beverages are permitted in laboratory areas.
- The student appropriately disposes of sharps into sharps containers and biohazard materials into biohazard bags/containers.

4) **The student correctly prepares, labels, packages, and stores samples for diagnostic laboratory examination.**
   - The student prepares and processes laboratory samples appropriately based on a correct understanding of the use of such samples in diagnostic tests.
   - The student demonstrates accurate labelling of diagnostic samples.
   - The student handles, packages, and stores diagnostic samples in a manner that ensures the maximum accuracy of results and is in accordance with laboratory guidelines.

6.2 Diagnostic Laboratory Procedures

5) **The student correctly determines the physical properties of urine samples.**
   - The student explains the effects of time and temperature on a urine sample and examines the urine sample at the correct temperature and in a timely manner.
   - The student accurately describes the color, clarity, and odor of the sample, using appropriate terminology.
   - The student correctly defines and displays understanding of the diagnostic significance of urine specific gravity. The student also correctly explains the terms *hyposthenuric, isosthenuric,* and *hypersthenuric* and their diagnostic significance.

- The student properly uses the refractometer to accurately measure the urine specific gravity, cleaning it properly after each use. The student frequently checks the calibration of the refractometer and correctly recalibrates it as needed.
- The student describes the significance of the color, clarity, odor, and specific gravity of the urine sample as they relate to the clinical condition.
- The student demonstrates understanding of reagent strips used to determine the chemical properties of urine. The student uses reagent strips properly, reading results accurately and in a timely manner. The student displays awareness that, depending on the species being tested, false positive and false negative results regarding the presence of cellular elements in urine may occur; therefore, these results should be verified with microscopic sediment analysis.
- The student properly prepares urine sediment for microscopic examination. Using correct microscopic technique, the student accurately identifies red blood cells, white blood cells, crystals, casts, artifacts, and other cellular elements, using experience and reference books.
- The student explains the significance of the results of the microscopic analysis as they relate to the clinical condition.

6) **The student demonstrates knowledge of how to accurately determine the hemoglobin concentration of a complete blood count (CBC).**
   - The student correctly explains the difference between plasma and serum and the appropriate methods to obtain plasma and serum.
   - The student correctly defines the term *hemoglobin* and correctly describes the structure and physiological functions of hemoglobin and the clinical relevance of the hemoglobin concentration.
   - The student displays knowledge of the appropriate blood sample tube and

anticoagulant for obtaining an accurate hemoglobin concentration.

- The student demonstrates the ability to accurately calculate the hemoglobin concentration.
- The student correctly explains the relationship between the hemoglobin concentration and the hematocrit (HCT). The student displays the ability to estimate the HCT based on the hemoglobin concentration.

7) **The student demonstrates correct methodology for obtaining a packed cell volume (PCV).**
- The student correctly explains the difference between plasma and serum.
- The student correctly defines the term *packed cell volume* and correctly explains its clinical relevance.
- The student displays awareness that, although the terms PCV and hematocrit (HCT) often are used interchangeably in the clinical setting, the HCT is a value calculated by automatic analyzers whereas the PCV is directly measured manually.
- The student uses the appropriate blood sample tube and anticoagulant for obtaining an accurate HCT.
- The student demonstrates the proper use of the microhematocrit tube and centrifuge to obtain a PCV.
- The student observes and makes note of the characteristics of the plasma, including color and turbidity.
- The student correctly measures the PCV, recognizes normal and abnormal values, and explains the clinical relevance.

8) **The student demonstrates correct methodology for determining the total protein concentration.**
- The student correctly explains the difference between plasma and serum.
- The student correctly explains the difference in the major protein constituents of plasma versus serum and describes the physiological functions and clinical relevance of each.

- The student uses the appropriate blood sample tube and anticoagulant to obtain the total protein concentration.
- The student demonstrates the proper use of the microhematocrit tube and centrifuge to obtain the total protein concentration.
- The student observes and makes note of the characteristics of the plasma, including color and turbidity.
- The student properly uses a refractometer to obtain the total protein concentration and properly cleans the refractometer after use.
- The student demonstrates understanding of the importance of evaluating PCV and total protein together to aid in the assessment of certain clinical conditions such as dehydration, hemorrhage, and hemolysis.

9) **The student demonstrates correct methodology for obtaining a white blood cell count.**
- The student correctly explains the difference between plasma and serum.
- The student correctly describes the general physiological functions of white blood cells and the clinical relevance of a white blood cell count.
- The student describes the various automated and manual methods by which a white blood cell count can be obtained, including the advantages and disadvantages of each. For example, the student correctly identifies that the white blood cell count from automated analyzers is more accurate because the automated analyzer counts thousands of cells (Samples, 2022).
- The student uses the appropriate blood sample tube and anticoagulant for obtaining a white blood cell count.
- The student demonstrates proper use of the microhematocrit tube and centrifuge to obtain the buffy coat.
- The student correctly identifies the constituents of a buffy coat.

- The student observes and makes note of the characteristics of the buffy coat.
- The student demonstrates the ability to properly prepare and stain a blood smear.
- The student correctly describes the regions of the blood smear and identifies the monolayer as the appropriate region of the blood smear to obtain a white blood cell count as well as observe the morphology of the white blood cells.
- The student demonstrates proper use of the microscope as well as the proper technique when evaluating a blood smear.
- The student accurately determines the white blood cell count.

10) **The student demonstrates correct methodology for obtaining a red blood cell count.**
   - The student correctly explains the difference between plasma and serum.
   - The student correctly describes the general physiological functions of red blood cells and clinical relevance of a red blood cell count.
   - The student correctly explains the difference between the packed cell volume (PCV) and the red blood cell count.
   - The student describes the various automated and manual methods by which a red blood cell count can be obtained, including the advantages and disadvantages of each. For example, the student correctly identifies that the red blood cell count from automated analyzers is more accurate because the automated analyzer counts thousands of cells (Samples, 2022).
   - The student uses the appropriate blood sample tube and anticoagulant for obtaining a red blood cell count.
   - The student demonstrates the ability to properly prepare and stain a blood smear.
   - The student correctly describes the regions of the blood smear and identifies the monolayer as the appropriate region of the blood smear to obtain a red blood cell count as well as observe the morphology of the red blood cells.

- The student demonstrates proper use of the microscope as well as the proper technique when evaluating a blood smear. The student accurately determines the red blood cell count.

11) **The student uses proper methodology to prepare blood films, showing proficiency in staining them with a variety of techniques.**
   - The student correctly prepares blood smears of appropriate length, width, and density.
   - The student shows familiarity with various stains and their appropriate applications.
   - The student correctly identifies the different regions of a properly prepared blood smear.
   - The student uses proper technique to stain blood films.

12) **The student demonstrates correct methodology for performing a leukocyte differential and accurately distinguishes between normal and abnormal cells.**
   - The student demonstrates the ability to properly prepare and stain a blood smear.
   - The student correctly describes the regions of the blood smear and identifies the monolayer as the appropriate region of the blood smear to observe the morphology of the white blood cells.
   - The student demonstrates proper use of the microscope as well as the proper technique when evaluating a blood smear.
   - The student evaluates the condition and state of all cells on the blood smear.
   - The student accurately identifies types of leukocytes, demonstrating understanding of species differences.
   - The student accurately differentiates between normal and abnormal cells and correctly explains the clinical relevance of commonly seen morphological changes.
   - The student performs a count of 100 leukocytes for the differential and accurately determines relative counts for each white cell type.

- The student accurately calculates the absolute count for each white blood cell type.
- The student displays understanding of the clinical significance of abnormal counts of each type of leukocyte.

13) **The student correctly assesses the morphology of erythrocytes and accurately distinguishes between normal and abnormal cells.**

- The student demonstrates the ability to properly prepare and stain a blood smear.
- The student correctly describes the regions of the blood smear and identifies the monolayer as the appropriate region of the blood smear to observe the morphology of the red blood cells.
- The student demonstrates proper use of the microscope as well as the proper technique when evaluating a blood smear.
- The student correctly evaluates red blood cells for morphological differences, demonstrating understanding of species differences. The student accurately identifies rouleaux formation, spherocytes, poikilocytes, macrocytes, microcytes, anisocytosis, polychromasia, and other red blood cell morphologies.
- The student accurately differentiates between normal and abnormal cells and distinguishes changes due to disease from those due to artifact or mechanical causes. The student correctly identifies inclusions such as Howell–Jolly bodies and Heinz bodies, as well as parasites, such as *Babesia* spp. and hemotropic *Mycoplasma* spp.
- The student demonstrates understanding of the diagnostic importance of erythrocyte morphology.

14) **The student demonstrates correct methodology for estimating thrombocyte numbers.**

- The student correctly describes some of the species differences in platelet counts

and appearance, as well as how these species differences affect the ability to obtain an accurate platelet count.

- The student demonstrates understanding of the importance of confirming platelet counts from an automated analyzer with a manual platelet count estimation on a blood smear.
- The student demonstrates the ability to properly prepare and stain a blood smear.
- The student correctly describes the regions of the blood smear and identifies the monolayer as the appropriate region of the blood smear to obtain an estimated platelet count.
- The student demonstrates proper use of the microscope as well as the proper technique when evaluating a blood smear.
- The student utilizes proper technique to perform estimated platelet counts on blood films, ensuring to check the edges of the monolayer for platelets and platelet clumping. The student accurately calculates estimated total platelet counts.
- The student displays knowledge of the diagnostic importance of platelet counts.

15) **The student accurately determines absolute values of leukocytes.**

- The student accurately calculates absolute values of leukocytes based on the relative percentages and total white blood cell count.
- The student demonstrates understanding of the diagnostic significance of absolute values of leukocytes.

16) **The student demonstrates proper methodology for performing corrected white blood cell counts due to the presence of other nucleated cells.**

- The student demonstrates the ability to correctly identify nucleated cells on a properly prepared and stained blood smear.
- The student explains the clinical significance of the presence of other nucleated cells in various species. For example, the nucleated red blood cell is normal in

birds. In dogs and cats, however, the presence of nucleated red blood cells is abnormal and may be clinically significant.

- The student demonstrates understanding of the necessity for performing a corrected white blood cell count due to the presence of other nucleated cells.
- The student accurately calculates the corrected white blood cell count.

17) **The student correctly determines red blood cell indices.**

- The student demonstrates knowledge of the diagnostic meaning of red blood cell indices, including mean corpuscular volume (MCV), mean corpuscular hemoglobin (MCH), mean corpuscular hemoglobin concentration (MCHC), and reticulocyte count.
- The student demonstrates the correct methodology for performing a reticulocyte count by counting 1000 red blood cells, correctly identifying reticulocytes, and accurately determining the relative percentage of reticulocytes.
- The student demonstrates an understanding that reticulocyte counts should be interpreted in light of the degree of anemia present and accurately calculates a corrected reticulocyte count.
- The student correctly calculates MCV, MCH, and MCHC.
- The student correctly differentiates normal versus abnormal values for RBC indices and explains the clinical significance of abnormalities.

18) **The student participates in correctly performing at least one of the following tests of blood coagulation: buccal mucosal bleeding time, activated clotting time (ACT), prothrombin time (PT), partial thromboplastin time (PTT), or fibrinogen assay.**

- The student demonstrates knowledge of the diagnostic significance of blood coagulation tests (e.g., buccal mucosal

bleeding time is used to assess primary hemostasis).

- The student explains the proper procedure for performing the blood coagulation test in which they were participating.
- The student appropriately participates in performing a coagulation test.
- The student accurately differentiates between normal versus abnormal results and correctly explains the clinical significance of abnormal results.

19) **The student demonstrates correct methodology for performing blood chemistry tests, including, but not limited to, urea nitrogen, glucose, and common enzymes.**

- The student correctly describes the difference between plasma and serum and explains why blood chemistry tests are performed on serum.
- The student shows awareness that certain in-house blood chemistry analyzers use plasma to perform blood chemistry tests and correctly uses plasma to perform blood chemistry tests when indicated.
- The student demonstrates understanding of the diagnostic significance of common blood chemistry tests.
- The student correctly performs blood chemistry tests.
- The student accurately differentiates between normal and abnormal results and explains the clinical significance of abnormal results.

20) **The student demonstrates correct methodology for performing serologic assays, including ELISA and slide/card agglutination tests.**

- The student displays understanding of the relevant physiology of immunology.
- The student demonstrates understanding of immunological principles underlying serological tests.
- The student shows understanding of the diagnostic importance of serological tests.

- The student properly performs and correctly interprets snap tests.
- The student properly performs and correctly interprets slide/card agglutination tests.
- The student displays the ability to differentiate between normal and abnormal results and explains their clinical significance.

21) **The student accurately identifies adult and immature stages of *Dirofilaria* spp. and *Acanthocheilonema* spp. (formerly *Dipetalonema* spp.).**
- The student correctly describes the heartworm life cycle.
- The student accurately differentiates microfilaria of *Dirofilaria* spp. from *Acanthocheilonema* spp. (formerly *Dipetalonema* spp.).
- The student demonstrates understanding of the clinical significance of the presence of *Dirofilaria* versus *Acanthocheilonema*.

22) **The student displays knowledge of how to detect the presence of mites and correctly identifies mites.**
- The student demonstrates knowledge of the clinical signs of different types of mite infestations and the clinical significance of each.
- The student shows knowledge of the zoonotic potential of mite infestation.
- The student displays knowledge of the proper procedure for detecting the presence of ear mites, including how to correctly take the sample from the ear and prepare the slide for microscopic examination.
- The student demonstrates knowledge of the proper procedures for detecting mites that burrow into the skin and mites that come from hair follicles, including the correct skin scrape techniques for *Sarcoptes* versus *Demodex* spp. The student shows knowledge of how to prepare the slide for microscopic evaluation. Using appropriate

microscopic technique, the student accurately identifies *Sarcoptes* and *Demodex* mites.
- The student shows awareness of how to detect *Sarcoptes* and *Demodex* mites or ova in fecal flotation. The student shows awareness that demodicosis, especially in cats, may be diagnosed via fecal flotation due to grooming behavior (Companion Animal Parasite Council, 2019).
- The student demonstrates knowledge of how to detect the presence of mites living on the skin surface or hair, such as *Cheyletiella*, using a fine-tooth flea comb and/or cellophane tape methods. The student shows knowledge of how to correctly prepare the slide for microscopic examination. The student accurately identifies *Cheyletiella*.

23) **The student displays knowledge of the proper procedure to detect the presence of lice and correctly identifies lice.**
- The student demonstrates familiarity with the life cycle of lice and differentiates between chewing (biting) versus sucking lice.
- The student shows awareness of routes of transmission (direct contact, fomites) and clinical signs of lice infestation.
- The student demonstrates knowledge of the proper procedure for detecting the presence of adult or nymphal lice and/or nits, including how to correctly collect nymphal/adult lice and/or nits. The student shows knowledge of how to prepare the slide for microscopic examination. The student demonstrates knowledge of how to correctly identify lice with microscopic examination.

24) **The student displays knowledge of the proper procedure to detect the presence of ticks and correctly identifies ticks.**
- The student shows knowledge of the basic tick structure (body parts).

- The student demonstrates knowledge of the role of ticks as vectors in the transmission of disease.
- The student displays knowledge of common tick-borne diseases, their clinical signs, the clinical relevance to an individual patient, and appropriate treatment.
- The student correctly identifies species of ticks acting as vectors for common infectious diseases, including, but not limited to, *Ixodes* spp. (*Borrelia burgdorferi*, Lyme disease), *Rhipicephalus sanguineous* (babesiosis, ehrlichiosis), *Dermacentor andersoni* and *Dermacentor variabilis* (Rocky Mountain Spotted Fever), etc.
- The student shows knowledge of how to properly inspect an animal for the presence of ticks, including those that may be hidden. The student demonstrates knowledge of how to correctly remove and dispose of ticks.
- The student demonstrates knowledge of how to correctly identify ticks with microscopic examination.

25) **The student displays knowledge of the proper procedures to detect the presence of fleas and correctly identifies fleas.**
- The student correctly identifies fleas, including, but not limited to, *Ctenocephalides felis*, and shows knowledge of their life cycles.
- The student shows knowledge of the role of fleas in carrying and transmitting infectious diseases, such as *Dipylidium caninum*.
- The student displays knowledge of common diseases associated with fleas, their clinical signs, the clinical relevance to an individual patient, and appropriate treatment.
- The student demonstrates knowledge of the common clinical signs of flea infestation and flea allergy dermatitis (FAD).

- The student displays knowledge of how to properly inspect an animal for the presence of fleas and/or flea dirt.

26) **The student displays knowledge of the proper procedures to detect the presence of flies and correctly identifies flies.**
- The student correctly identifies flies and shows familiarity with their life cycles.
- The student shows knowledge of common clinical signs of fly bites as well as clinical signs of fly larvae that invade the body. The student demonstrates cognizance of the role of flies as vectors for infectious disease.
- The student displays knowledge of common diseases associated with flies, their clinical signs, the clinical relevance to an individual patient, and appropriate treatment.
- The student accurately identifies maggot infestation.
- The student shows knowledge that a skin lesion with a central pore is a sign of *Cuterebra* infestation.

27) **The student uses correct methodology to perform heartworm diagnostic procedures, including the antigen kit, direct (examination of blood), and the modified Knotts test.**
- The student displays knowledge of the immunological basis of the heartworm antigen test.
- The student shows cognizance of the potential for false negative results on the antigen test and why they occur.
- The student demonstrates knowledge of the importance of timing the antigen kit test based on the heartworm life cycle and prepatent period, in order to maximize accuracy of results.
- The student properly performs and accurately interprets the results of the heartworm antigen test kit.
- The student displays knowledge of how to detect microfilaria by observing their movement beneath the buffy coat in a

- The student displays knowledge of the canine estrous cycle and common pathogens of the canine vagina.
- The student shows familiarity with indications for performing canine vaginal smears.
- The student participates in obtaining canine vaginal smears.
- The student participates in preparing the smear for microscopic evaluation.
- The student accurately evaluates canine vaginal smears.

45) **The student participates in performing a necropsy on a non-preserved animal, using all available precautions to minimize the risk of zoonotic disease.**

- The student demonstrates anatomical knowledge, including the ability to identify normal versus abnormal anatomy pertinent to postmortem examination.
- The student demonstrates awareness of the risk of infectious disease from tissue and/or fluids of deceased animals, regardless of whether the patient was diagnosed with such disease.
- When handling necropsy specimens, the student shows the ability to apply knowledge of the transmission routes of zoonotic diseases.
- The student displays awareness of the extreme importance of personal protective equipment in performing a necropsy, including, but not limited to, full-body aprons, nitrile gloves, masks, and appropriate footwear.
- The student shows the ability to determine which tissue/fluid samples might be of greatest importance based on knowledge of the patient's diagnosis at the time of death. At the same time, the student demonstrates understanding that samples from all major organs and other tissue, if diseased (e.g., oral cavity) and/or requested by veterinarian and/or pathologist, should be harvested, as should relevant fluids (e.g., peritoneal, pleural, blood, ocular globe, etc.). The

student also demonstrates knowledge that when collecting samples care should be taken to include any lesion, transitional tissue, and normal tissue.
- The student displays knowledge of and participates in the proper procedure for performing a postmortem examination on a non-preserved animal, including appropriate recording of diagnostic information in the medical record.

46) **The student correctly obtains, stores, and ships specimens, following procedures required by the diagnostic laboratory.**

- The student shows awareness of the importance of collecting multiple samples from major organs and, when relevant, entire organs, such as kidneys or lymph nodes.
- The student displays knowledge that samples must be large enough to be sliced to allow slide preparation.
- The student displays knowledge that fluid samples should be retained either in capped, sterile syringes or in sterile vials as directed by the pathologist.
- The student displays knowledge that 10% neutral, buffered formalin is used for fixation of most tissue types and there should be a minimum of 10 parts of formalin to 1 part of tissue (Samples, 2022).
- The student displays knowledge of proper procedures for the safe handling of formalin containers. The student demonstrates awareness of potential risks of exposure to formalin that may occur while filling jars and placing samples, particularly its carcinogenic risks.
- The student correctly places tissue samples in formalin jars of appropriate size, properly labeling them.
- The student displays knowledge of how to correctly gather all samples from the patient, either storing them for in-house use or packaging them according to requirements of the diagnostic laboratory. The student shows understanding that proper packaging is directed at preventing

spillage or breakage and making certain the shipping box is appropriately labeled (e.g., indicating that contents are biological samples, indicating the top of the package, and, when appropriate, any biohazard potential).

- The student wears nitrile gloves when handling specimens, even when they are handling closed containers.
- The student demonstrates knowledge of how to properly package and ship clinical specimens as well as the ability to participate in specimen handling and preparation. The student shows awareness that individual courier companies should be contacted regarding specific packaging requirements since these may differ from one courier to another.

47) **The student displays knowledge of how to safely handle rabies suspects and specimens.**

- The student demonstrates knowledge of the pathogenesis of rabies and the stages of the disease in the affected animal.
- The student displays knowledge of rabies transmission, as well as state and/or local regulations governing the handling of rabies suspects and specimens.
- The student shows awareness that any mammal that dies of unknown cause, as well as any animal that displayed signs of rabies in life, is treated as a rabies suspect.
- The student exhibits understanding that rabies is a zoonotic, reportable, and fatal disease to animals and humans. Therefore, any person working with live or dead mammals should be immunized against rabies.

- The student displays understanding of state protocols that must be followed, including proper procedures for obtaining recommended human postexposure treatment, if there is any question regarding accidental exposure to tissues from a rabies suspect.
- The student displays knowledge of PPE that must be worn when obtaining samples from rabies suspects, including, but not limited to, face shields, waterproof gowns, full-length sleeves, and double gloves. The student shows knowledge that, after handling any samples from rabies suspects, all PPE must be shed and either disposed of in a biohazard container or submitted in a biohazard container to the laboratory for appropriate decontamination.
- The student shows knowledge that rabies can be definitively diagnosed only in isolated central nervous system tissue, particularly brain tissue. In small animal cases where the primary differential diagnosis is rabies, the entire head is removed from the body and shipped to the appropriate diagnostic laboratory. The student shows knowledge that the head should be shipped refrigerated (and never frozen); however, the appropriate state diagnostic laboratory should be contacted for specific instructions, since these may vary from state to state.
- The student displays knowledge that for large animal rabies suspects, some states require removal of the brain prior to submission to the diagnostic laboratory. Therefore, the appropriate state laboratory should be contacted for specific instructions (Samples, 2022).

References

American Heartworm Society. (2020a) *Current Canine Guidelines for the Prevention, Diagnosis, and Management of Heartworm (Dirofilaria immitis) Infection in Dogs.*

Retrieved June 7, 2023 from American Heartworm Society, https://d3ft8sckhnqim2.cloudfront.net/images/pdf/2018_AHS_Canine_Guidelines_rev_7-25-19.pdf?1564157216

American Heartworm Society. (2020b) *Summary of the Current Feline Guidelines for the Prevention, Diagnosis, and Management of Heartworm (Dirofilaria immitis) Infection in Cats*. Retrieved June 7, 2023 from American Heartworm Society, https://d3ft8sckhnqim2. cloudfront.net/images/pdf/2020_AHS_ Feline_Guidelines_Summary_11_12. pdf?1605556516

Clinical and Laboratory Standards Institute. (2023). *Performance Standards for Disk and Dilution Susceptibility Tests for Bacteria Isolated from Animals* (6th ed.) Wayne, PA: CLSI standard VET01S Clinical and Laboratory Standards Institute.

Companion Animal Parasite Council (2019). *Demodex* spp. Retrieved November 19, 2023 from Companion Animal Parasite Council. https://capcvet.org/guidelines/demodex/.

Hendrix, C. M. and Robinson, E. (2023). *Diagnostic Parasitology for Veterinary Technicians*, 6th e. (p. 281). St. Louis: Elsevier.

Samples, O. M. (2022). Basic necropsy procedures. In *McCurnin's Clinical Textbook for Veterinary Technicians and Nurses*, 10th e. (ed. J. M. Bassert, A. D. Beal, O. M. Samples), 480–499. St. Louis: Elsevier.

Schenkel, L. E., Timperman, S., Buell, L.J., Duffelmeyer-Kramer, J., Sturtz, R. E., and Douglas, D. (2017). Clinical laboratory procedures. In *Assessing Essential Skills of Veterinary Technology Students*, 3rd e. (ed. L. J. Buell, L. E. Schenkel, and S. Timperman), 25–35. Ames: John Wiley & Sons, Inc.

Sirois, M., and Hendrix, C. M. (2020). *Laboratory Procedures for Veterinary Technicians*, 7th e. (pp. 240, 258). St. Louis: Elsevier.

7

Radiography
Sandra Lynn Bertholf, MS, LVT

1) **The student demonstrates and follows recommended procedures for radiation safety.**
   - The student acts in accordance with rules and regulations contained in Ionizing Radiation – Toxic and Hazardous Substances – Occupational Safety and Health Standards (United States Department of Labor, 1996).
   - The student shows awareness that the following individuals are not permitted in the radiography room during exposure: those less than 18 years of age, pregnant women, and unnecessary personnel.
   - The student shows awareness that manually restraining an animal for radiography should only be undertaken when all other forms of restraint are impossible or would be a significant health/safety risk to the patient. The student displays awareness that the best safety measure is refraining from being in the radiography room during exposure.
   - The student demonstrates knowledge of potential health dangers associated with radiation, maximum permissible doses (MPD) per year (whole body, individual tissues, and lens of eye), and the lifetime cumulative effects of radiation.
   - The student displays familiarity with the various types of personal protective equipment (PPE) and their proper applications.

   - The student correctly wears appropriate PPE, including, but not limited to, lead apron, gloves, thyroid shield, badge, and lead safety glasses for every exposure. In addition, the student displays awareness that all PPE must be worn correctly. For example, gloves must be worn properly; laying gloves on top of hands and arms is unacceptable.
   - The student demonstrates understanding of the necessity of personal monitoring devices (dosimeter badges) and their purpose.
   - The student properly stores PPE. Gloves should be stored vertically on holders or lying flat with the ends propped open. Thyroid shields should be laid flat and lead safety glasses should be stored in a manner that prevents scratching or damage. Lead aprons should never be folded but instead draped over a rack.
   - The student displays awareness that PPE should be inspected routinely, radiographed at least yearly to detect defects, and the results properly documented. Defective PPE should be discarded and replaced.
   - The student wears their dosimeter badge correctly, positioning it outside the apron at the thyroid gland level. The student shows awareness that the dosimeter badge should be worn when in the

Assessing Essential Skills of Veterinary Technology Students, Fourth Edition. Edited by Lisa E. Schenkel, Amanda Colón, Sandra Lynn Bertholf, Sabrina Timperman, and Laurie J. Buell.
© 2024 John Wiley & Sons, Inc. Published 2024 by John Wiley & Sons, Inc.
Companion website: www.wiley.com/go/Schenkel/AssessingEssentialSkillsofVeterinaryTechnologyStudents4e

facility. When not in use, the student makes certain to store the dosimeter badge in a place protected from exposure to radiation (including sunlight), heat, or chemicals.

- The student displays knowledge of the limitations of PPE. In particular, the student demonstrates understanding that PPE helps provide protection from scatter radiation only and does not protect against direct radiation. The student shows awareness that at no time should any part of their body be within the primary X-ray beam, even if wearing PPE.
- The student demonstrates awareness of the importance of using proper collimation to reduce scatter radiation, thereby decreasing radiation exposure for personnel involved.
- The student displays good judgement and takes all appropriate steps to minimize radiation exposure of personnel and patients.

2) **The student displays knowledge of how effective radiographic quality control procedures help to ensure production of diagnostic images.**

- The student correctly defines the terms *density* and *contrast* and explains how they affect radiographic quality.
- The student demonstrates knowledge of how to evaluate whether radiographs are of diagnostic quality. The student displays understanding of whether proper contrast and density have been achieved and demonstrates knowledge of how to adjust settings appropriately to acquire a quality image.
- The student displays awareness of how to record or appropriately log radiographic technique to help ensure continued quality images for that patient.
- The student displays knowledge of artifacts, their causes, and how to correct them. For example, the student shows awareness that lack of contrast may be due to a light leak, radiation fog (exposure to undesired radiation), storage fog (heat and excess humidity), chemical fog (expired chemicals or excessive chemical temperature), expired film, improper technique, etc.

3) **The student demonstrates knowledge of how to correctly use a radiographic technique chart.**

- The student displays awareness that every individual X-ray machine, whether conventional or digital, should have its own technique chart based on its unique features and that multiple technique charts may be necessary (such as tabletop vs. Bucky) (Brown, M. and Brown, L., 2022).
- The student demonstrates the ability to use a technique chart to select correct settings for individual animals, depending on tissue thickness and the body part being radiographed.
- The student displays understanding of how to carefully measure and position patients, and how to choose appropriate radiographic techniques (based on the technique chart) to minimize the need for repeat exposures.

4) **The student shows understanding of how to appropriately adjust radiographic techniques for exotic animal patients, including mice, rats, guinea pigs, lizards, and amphibians.**

- The student displays understanding that, for most exotic species, measurements are often not used to calculate exposure factors; rather, these are determined based on species and general size (Brown, M. and Brown, L., 2022).
- The student displays knowledge of normal exotic animal anatomy.
- The student displays understanding that correct patient positioning is often achieved using anatomical landmarks rather than palpation.
- The student shows awareness that positioning techniques for small rodents, lizards and amphibians differ depending

on the type of radiographic equipment being used. For example, when using conventional or computed radiography (CR) systems, the patient is directly positioned on the radiographic cassette. The student displays knowledge of appropriate techniques for the type of X-ray machine being used and how to adjust kVp to reflect the small size of the patient (Brown, M. and Brown, L., 2022).

- The student displays understanding that while ideal positioning is often achieved by using sedation or anesthesia, patient status may preclude that option (Brown, M. and Brown, L., 2022).
- The student displays awareness of the proper restraint techniques and equipment used in exotic species.
- The student displays understanding that when using conventional X-ray machine, using the fastest film-screen combinations and/or minimizing exposure time will aid in avoiding a blurry image due to movement.
- For lizards and amphibians, the student demonstrates awareness that when using a conventional X-ray machine or a CR digital system, lateral radiographs should be taken using a horizontal beam at peak inspiration, since placing these species in lateral position distorts the lungs and diaphragm (Brown, M. and Brown, L., 2022).

5) **The student demonstrates the ability to properly position dogs, cats, and horses/ponies/donkeys/mules for radiographic studies.**
- The student shows awareness of the correct views to properly visualize the area of interest.
- The student demonstrates knowledge of pertinent canine and feline anatomy.
- The student correctly measures and positions dogs and cats for radiographic studies.
- The student is able to define and properly demonstrate positioning terms such as lateral, ventrodorsal, dorsoventral, dorsopalmar, dorsoplantar, and craniocaudal.

- The student correctly uses positioning aids and restraints, such as wedges, sandbags, tape, ties, cotton rolls, foam or plastic troughs, and so on, to position patients for diagnostic imaging.
- The student demonstrates proper patient handling and is aware of safety concerns associated with chemical and physical restraints, recognizing that the safety of both the patient and personnel are of the highest priority.
- The student displays knowledge of pertinent equine anatomy.
- The student demonstrates awareness of how beam distance and positional aspects affect equine radiography.
- The student shows knowledge of the potential for their exposure to radiation when operating hand-held and/or portable radiographic equipment.
- The student demonstrates proper equine restraint techniques and is aware of safety precautions in handling injured horses, recognizing that the safety of both patient and personnel are of the highest priority.
- The student properly prepares an equine patient for a radiographic procedure. For example, when obtaining diagnostic images of the hoof, horseshoes should be removed and the lateral sulci of the frog packed with an appropriate material.
- The student demonstrates the ability to position the equine distal limb in a series of oblique, lateral, dorsopalmar, dorsoplantar, and/or proximodistal ("skyline" view) positions.

6) **The student demonstrates the ability to position live animals or intubated non-preserved specimens and to use dental radiographic equipment to produce intra-oral full mouth dental radiographs of the dog and cat that are of diagnostic quality.**
- The student demonstrates appropriate knowledge of the anatomy of the oral cavity.
- The student disconnects the anesthetic circuit from the ET tube when repositioning

the patient to prevent tracheal injury. For example, when changing patient position from dorsal to ventral recumbency, the ET tube should not be connected to the anesthetic circuit. The student reconnects the anesthetic circuit and makes certain the ET tube is correctly positioned and inflated once the patient is repositioned.

- The student properly positions the patient, film/sensor, and beam in the appropriate location to create a diagnostic image. For example, the student utilizes the parallel technique only for radiographing mandibular premolars and molars. The bisecting angle technique is utilized for radiographing all other teeth.
- The student uses the correct film/sensor and placement.
- The student properly adjusts the image by changing exposure time.
- The student demonstrates the proper use of sandbags, bite blocks, V-shaped troughs, gauze, or any other type of positioning device needed to assist in increasing stability and correct placement.
- The student properly acquires diagnostic quality images of all four quadrants of the mouth.

7) **The student properly labels, files, and stores radiographic film studies.**

- The student stores film images appropriately. For example, the student displays knowledge of the need to protect film from temperature extremes, ionizing radiation, and high humidity.
- The student displays awareness that expired film should not be used because it will decrease image quality.
- The student properly handles both unexposed and exposed film, for example, handling film by the corners only.
- The student permanently labels images with required information including, but not limited to, patient identification, client identification, date, hospital and/or veterinarian's name, body part being radiographed, and positioning.

- The student files radiographic film studies correctly and in an organized manner.

8) **The student properly labels, files, and stores radiographic digital studies.**

- The student stores digital images appropriately. For example, the student displays knowledge of the need to archive images on a computer and that images must be stored in more than one place due to the potential for data loss. Storage of digital images may be duplicated by cloud storage or offsite data storage companies.
- The student attaches digital images to the patient's medical record in accordance with the digital medical record system used by the facility.
- The student enters all required information including, but not limited to, patient identification, client identification, date, hospital, and/or veterinarian's name, body part being radiographed, and positioning, into the digital system prior to obtaining radiograph.

9) **The student demonstrates understanding of how to properly complete radiographic logs, reports, files, and records.**

- The student displays understanding of how to properly log and file radiographic studies.
- The student demonstrates understanding of the required information for a radiographic log based on the system used by the facility.
- The student shows knowledge of how to correctly record information of the radiographic study in the patient's medical record.

10) **The student participates in utilizing either positive or negative contrast agents in performing a gastrointestinal (GI) series, pneumocystogram, intravenous pyelogram, or other radiographic contrast study.**

- The student demonstrates knowledge of the pertinent anatomy to properly perform a GI series, pneumocystogram, intravenous pyelogram, or other radiographic contrast study.

- The student displays knowledge of various contrast agents, their uses, and correct routes and sites of administration.
- The student correctly calculates doses of contrast agents.
- The student shows awareness of potential common adverse effects associated with various contrast studies and contrast agents. For example, dehydration should be corrected before performing an intravenous pyelogram to decrease the risk of potential renal damage.
- The student closely monitors patients during and following a contrast study.
- The student shows knowledge of how to accurately time and properly label images when performing a GI series or intravenous pyelogram.
- The student shows knowledge of how to properly use air as a contrast medium when performing a negative contrast study such as a pneumocystogram.

11) **The student participates in correctly performing radiographic screening for canine hip dysplasia (CHD).**
- The student displays knowledge of normal canine hip anatomy and appropriate anatomic landmarks to correctly perform radiographic screening for CHD.
- The student demonstrates knowledge of the multifactorial pathophysiology of canine hip dysplasia, including its genetic roots, the influence of nutritional factors, and its prevalence in certain breeds.
- The student explains the importance of only breeding dogs with acceptable certification but is aware that this does not guarantee that offspring will not have CHD.
- The student is aware of the minimum age requirement for accurate CHD evaluation in relation to the specific technique being used.
- The student shows familiarity with Orthopedic Foundation for Animals (OFA) and PennHIP techniques, their relative advantages and disadvantages, and the different requirements for each.
- The student displays knowledge of how to properly position a dog for radiographic evaluation for CHD, explaining why proper positioning is crucial and how improper positioning can lead to a nondiagnostic image.
- The student is aware that general anesthesia is required for accurate PennHIP evaluation and that deep sedation or general anesthesia is recommended for accurate OFA evaluation.
- The student differentiates between diagnostic and non-diagnostic images. The student shows familiarity with rating scales for OFA and PennHIP techniques.

12) **The student displays knowledge of the correct care and maintenance of radiographic equipment and is able to recognize when it is defective.**
- The student demonstrates knowledge of basic principles regarding how radiographic equipment operates.
- The student demonstrates awareness of the need for routine scheduled maintenance to ensure consistent quality diagnostic imaging and safety.
- The student demonstrates knowledge of how to properly identify defective radiographic equipment – for example, when the collimator light is nonfunctional and the proper field size cannot be assessed.
- The student recognizes when it is necessary for the manufacturer to service the equipment.
- The student demonstrates familiarity with common artifacts, their causes, and how to correct and prevent them.

References

Bertholf, S. and Timperman S. (2017). Radiography. In *Assessing Essential Skills of Veterinary Technology Students*, 3rd e. (ed. L. J. Buell, L. E. Schenkel, and S. Timperman), 59–62. Ames: John Wiley & Sons, Inc.

Brown, M. and Brown, L. (2022). *Lavin's Radiography for Veterinary Technicians*, 7th e. (pp. 68–81, 579–625). St Louis: Elsevier.

United States Department of Labor. (1996, June 20). Ionizing radiation. Retrieved June 22, 2023, from Occupational Safety and Health Administration. https://www.osha.gov/ionizing-radiation.

8

Laboratory Animal Care and Procedures
Nina Slivinsky, LVT, LATg

1) **The student displays understanding of the need for the use of laboratory animals in biomedical research.**
   - The student shows appreciation of the importance of upholding ethical, humane, and scientific standards in the use of laboratory animals.
   - The student explains the importance of the veterinary technician's/technologist's role in animal welfare as the provider of appropriate care of the laboratory animals.
   - The student demonstrates understanding of how to educate co-workers and other laboratory personnel appropriately and effectively on how to uphold the welfare of laboratory animals.

2) **The student displays working knowledge of federal, state, local, and institutional animal welfare regulations as they apply to laboratory animal research.**
   - The student demonstrates working knowledge of the content of the *Guide for the Care and Use of Laboratory Animals* (National Research Council, 2011).
   - The student demonstrates understanding of the importance of the Institutional Animal Care and Use Committee (IACUC) as it pertains to laboratory animal medicine and research (National Research Council, 2011; Bayne and Anderson, 2015).

   - The student displays understanding of the IACUC member's responsibilities and functions in research settings, which include (National Research Council, 2011; Bayne and Anderson, 2015):
     - Assessing facility operations and procedures
     - Reviewing research protocols
     - Ensuring institutional compliance
     - Reviewing methods to improve animal health and welfare
     - Supporting the 3 Rs (*replacement, reduction, refinement*), which constitute the backbone of all approved protocols and the animal use programs in research.

3) **The student correctly identifies and properly restrains rodents (mice, rats) and rabbits.**
   - The student correctly identifies and differentiates mice, rats, and rabbits.
   - The student correctly restrains adult and weanling mice by using one hand to grasp the base of the tail while the other hand is scruffing the neck (American Association of Laboratory Animal Science (AALAS), 2021; Suckow, Hashway, and Pritchett-Corning, 2023).
   - The student correctly restrains mice using rubber-tipped forceps by grasping the loose skin around the neck region or

Assessing Essential Skills of Veterinary Technology Students, Fourth Edition. Edited by Lisa E. Schenkel, Amanda Colón, Sandra Lynn Bertholf, Sabrina Timperman, and Laurie J. Buell.
© 2024 John Wiley & Sons, Inc. Published 2024 by John Wiley & Sons, Inc.
Companion website: www.wiley.com/go/Schenkel/AssessingEssentialSkillsofVeterinaryTechnologyStudents4e

close to the base of the tail (AALAS, 2021; Suckow, Hashway, and Pritchett-Corning, 2023).

- The student correctly restrains rats by using one hand to grab the base of the tail closest to the rump while placing the other hand over the back of the rat and simultaneously using the thumb and forefinger to press the forelegs near the head (AALAS, 2021; Champion, Calantropio-Covington, and Sirois, 2022).
- The student properly restrains rabbits, making certain to support their hindquarters. The student demonstrates knowledge of the rabbit's susceptibility to injury if improperly restrained, particularly its tendency to kick and sustain bone fractures. The student displays understanding that rabbits are never to be handled by the ears (AALAS 2021; Champion, Calantropio-Covington, and Sirois, 2022).
- The student demonstrates recognition and proper use of the various restraint devices used in laboratory animal medicine for rodents (mice, rats) and rabbits (AALAS, 2021; Champion, Calantropio-Covington, and Sirois, 2022; Suckow, Hashway, and Pritchett-Corning, 2023; Suckow and Schroeder, 2010).

4) **The student correctly determines the sex and demonstrates knowledge of the reproduction of rodents (mice, rats) and rabbits.**

- The student correctly identifies rodent gender via comparing the anogenital distance (distance between the genital papilla and anus) and the lack of grossly visible nipples in males (Champion, Calantropio-Covington, and Sirois, 2022).
- The student displays awareness that the doe (female rabbit) often has a large dewlap (skin fold that hangs around the neck) at the caudal mandibulocervical region (under the chin) and that the buck (male rabbit) lacks a dewlap (Champion, Calantropio-Covington, and Sirois, 2022).

- Based on accurate knowledge of anatomy, the student demonstrates the proper technique to sex a rabbit by using gentle pressure with the thumb and forefinger around the genital area to allow visibility of genitalia, while observing the genital opening (Champion, Calantropio-Covington, and Sirois, 2022).
- The student displays knowledge of estrous cycles, breeding characteristics, gestation periods, parturition, and litter sizes of mice, rats, and rabbits (Champion, Calantropio-Covington, and Sirois, 2022; Suckow and Schroeder, 2010). For example, based on accurate knowledge of physiology, the student displays understanding:
  - That female mice and rats are in estrus every 4–5 days, whereas rabbits are induced ovulators.
  - That the presence of a copulatory (vaginal) plug is an indication of mating in mice and rats.
  - That the gestation period for mice is 12–19 days, for rats it is 21–23 days, and for rabbits it is 31–32 days.
  - Of the definition of the Whitten effect.
  - That the doe is always taken to the buck's cage for mating.
  - That does pull fur from their dewlaps, chests, and abdomens to create nest boxes in preparation for kits (newborn rabbits).

5) **The student demonstrates proper handling of rodents (mice, rats) and rabbits**.

- The student correctly grasps and handles mouse pups by picking up a group of pups together, gently grasping the skin near and around their shoulder blades or by cupping hands around the body (AALAS, 2021; Champion, Calantropio-Covington, and Sirois, 2022).
- The student correctly handles adult/weanling mice using rubber-tipped forceps or fingertips by grasping the loose skin around the neck region or close to

the base of the tail (AALAS, 2021; Suckow, Hashway, and Pritchett-Corning, 2023).

- The student correctly handles adults/weanling rats by using one hand to grab the base of the tail closest to the rump while placing the other hand over the back of the rat and simultaneously using the thumb and forefinger to press the forelegs near the head (AALAS, 2021; Champion, Calantropio-Covington, and Sirois, 2022).
- The student correctly transports rats by placing a hand around the thorax and abdomen, taking care not to squeeze the thorax.
- The student safely and effectively picks up rabbits by using one hand to scruff the nape of the neck and the other hand to support the hindquarters (AALAS, 2021; Suckow and Schroeder, 2010). When carrying a rabbit long distances, the student demonstrates the ability to correctly restrain the rabbit with the rabbit's head nestled in the bend of the elbow and the hindquarters supported (Champion, Calantropio-Covington, and Sirois, 2022). Additionally, the student will demonstrate the proper use of transport carriers.

6) **The student shows knowledge of proper diets for laboratory rodents (mice, rats) and rabbits based on their unique nutritional requirements**.
- The student displays understanding of how their unique anatomy and physiology contributes to the nutritional requirements of mice, rats, and rabbits.
- The student shows knowledge that for adult laboratory rabbits, a good-quality, high-fiber diet should comprise the mainstay of the diet in order to prevent hairball formation and obesity. The student demonstrates understanding that although nutritional requirements may vary based on breed and life-stage, commercial nutritionally balanced rabbit pellets with free-choice timothy or grass hay will meet

the nutritional requirements of most rabbits and that supplemental foods such as raw carrots and other vegetables may be offered in limited amounts (AALAS, 2021; Champion, Calantropio-Covington, and Sirois, 2022).
- The student demonstrates knowledge that rabbits are coprophagic animals and consume cecotrophs (which are products of the cecum and provide necessary nutrients) directly from their anuses, usually at night (Champion, Calantropio-Covington, and Sirois, 2022).
- The student shows knowledge that a proper diet for adult rats and mice consists of commercial nutritionally balanced rat/rodent pellets which may vary in fat and protein content depending on study protocols (AALAS, 2021; Otto, Franklin, and Clifford, 2015; Whary et al., 2015).

7) **The student provides appropriate, species-specific food, water, and enrichment for rodents (mice, rats) and rabbits**
- The student checks daily to ensure that *ad lib* fresh water is provided in clean sipper tubes or bottles.
- For rats and mice, the student provides appropriate rodent pellets *ad lib* unless otherwise specified by the research IACUC protocol.
- For laboratory rabbits, the student provides appropriate rabbit pellets and timothy or grass hay *ad lib* and provides scheduled supplemental feed unless otherwise specified by the research IACUC protocol.
- The student displays knowledge of the purpose of enrichment given to mice and rats and provides appropriate enrichment, such as Nestlets, Nylabones®, Mouse Igloos®, Enviro-dri®, and housing huts.
- The student displays knowledge of the purpose of enrichment given to rabbits and provides appropriate enrichment, such as ropes, balls, Nylabones®, and nest boxes.

8) **The student displays knowledge of how to perform identification procedures in mice, rats, and rabbits.**
   - The student displays understanding of identification systems for mice, rats, and rabbits as well as which systems are appropriate for use in each species (AALAS, 2021; Champion, Calantropio-Covington, and Sirois, 2022; Suckow, Hashway, Pritchett-Corning, 2023; Suckow and Schroeder, 2010).
   - The student shows knowledge of how to perform identification procedures, including ear notching/punching/tagging, tattooing, and microchipping and applying permanent dye (AALAS, 2021; Champion, Calantropio-Covington, and Sirois, 2022; Suckow, Hashway, Pritchett-Corning, 2023).
   - The student displays awareness that toe clipping should only be performed on neonatal mice (AALAS, 2021; Suckow, Hashway, Pritchett-Corning, 2023).

9) **The student properly performs subcutaneous injections in mice, rats, and rabbits.**
   - The student demonstrates knowledge of the maximum volume that can be administered subcutaneously in each species (AALAS, 2021; Champion, Calantropio-Covington, and Sirois, 2022; Suckow, Hashway, Pritchett-Corning, 2023; Suckow and Schroeder, 2010).
   - With the animal properly restrained, the student correctly places the needle into the loose skin of the scruff (between the skin and underlying muscle in the hypodermis) and slowly injects the solution (AALAS, 2021; Champion, Calantropio-Covington, and Sirois, 2022; Suckow, Hashway, Pritchett-Corning, 2023; Suckow and Schroeder, 2010).

10) **The student participates in properly performing an intraperitoneal injection in the rat.**
   - The student demonstrates knowledge of the maximum volume that can be administered intraperitoneally to rats (AALAS, 2021; Champion, Calantropio-Covington, and Sirois, 2022).
   - The student displays knowledge of the anatomy of the peritoneal cavity of a rat and how that contributes to the location of the intraperitoneal injection.
   - The student shows understanding of the potential complications of peritoneal injections.
   - The student correctly describes how to administer drugs intraperitoneally in the rat, injecting lateral to midline into the caudal right quadrant of the abdomen (AALAS, 2021; Champion, Calantropio-Covington, and Sirois, 2022).
   - The student participates in correctly restraining the rat for intraperitoneal injection and/or performing the injection.

11) **The student participates in correctly collecting IV blood samples from the rat and the mouse.**
   - The student correctly describes how to obtain blood from the tail vein of the rat, using the "warm tail technique" to promote vasodilation (AALAS, 2021; Champion, Calantropio-Covington, and Sirois, 2022).
   - The student participates in properly restraining the rat for IV blood collection and/or performing venipuncture.
   - The student correctly describes how to obtain blood from the submandibular vein of a mouse (AALAS, 2021).
   - The student participates in properly restraining the mouse for IV blood collection and/or performing venipuncture.

12) **The student participates in correctly collecting IV blood samples from the rabbit.**
   - The student participates in properly obtaining blood samples from rabbits using the lateral/marginal ear vein, the lateral saphenous vein, and/or the central ear artery (AALAS, 2021; Champion, Calantropio-Covington, and Sirois, 2022).
   - The student displays awareness that sedation may be required for individual

rabbits, particularly if large amounts of blood must be collected (AALAS, 2021; Champion, Calantropio-Covington, and Sirois, 2022).

13) **The student participates in properly performing oral dosing in rats and mice.**

- The student demonstrates an understanding of the difference between oral gavaging and gastric gavaging.
- The student demonstrates knowledge of pertinent anatomy in rodents, including structures of the oral cavity, esophagus, and stomach (AALAS, 2021; Champion, Calantropio-Covington, and Sirois, 2022; Suckow, Hashway, Pritchett-Corning, 2023).
- The student shows awareness of potential dangers of administering oral medications to species that cannot vomit (AALAS, 2021; Champion, Calantropio-Covington, and Sirois, 2022; Suckow, Hashway, Pritchett-Corning, 2023).
- The student displays appreciation of the importance of measuring a sufficient distance from the mouth to the sternum so that the gavage tube is appropriately placed (AALAS, 2021).
- The student participates in properly inserting a gavage tube and administering drugs to rodents by this route (AALAS, 2021).
- The student demonstrates familiarity with dosing syringes, feeding tubes, and metal balling guns (AALAS, 2021; Champion, Calantropio-Covington, and Sirois, 2022; Suckow, Hashway, Pritchett-Corning, 2023).

14) **The student displays functional knowledge of anesthetic and recovery procedures in rats, mice, and rabbits**.

- In general, the student demonstrates basic knowledge of appropriate uses, major contraindications, common adverse effects, and appropriate routes and methods of administration for injectable and inhalant anesthetic, pre-anesthetic, and/or analgesic agents commonly used in rats, mice, and rabbits (Champion, Calantropio-Covington, and Sirois, 2022; Suckow, Hashway, Pritchett-Corning, 2023).
- The student demonstrates knowledge of how to administer an injectable agent to induce anesthesia in mice, rats, and rabbits and how to maintain anesthesia by administering an inhalant anesthetic via face mask or nose cone (AALAS, 2021; Champion, Calantropio-Covington, and Sirois, 2022; Suckow, Hashway, Pritchett-Corning, 2023).
- The student shows awareness that, in general, food and water should not be withheld prior to surgery in rats, mice, and rabbits (Champion, Calantropio-Covington, and Sirois, 2022).
- The student displays awareness of the need to apply ophthalmic lubricant in rodents and rabbits (Champion, Calantropio-Covington, and Sirois, 2022).
- The student displays knowledge of how to monitor anesthesia in rats, mice, and rabbits, properly checking respiratory and cardiovascular parameters, body temperature, muscle tone, and reflexes (e.g., palpebral, pedal, pinna, corneal, etc.) (Champion, Calantropio-Covington, and Sirois, 2022; Suckow, Hashway, Pritchett-Corning, 2023; Suckow and Schroeder, 2010).
- The student displays knowledge of how to recognize and address anesthetic overdose, hypothermia, hypotension, and other common anesthetic complications (Champion, Calantropio-Covington, and Sirois, 2022; Suckow, Hashway, Pritchett-Corning, 2023).
- The student demonstrates knowledge of appropriate thermoregulation devices (Suckow, Hashway, Pritchett-Corning, 2023; Suckow and Schroeder, 2010).
- The student demonstrates knowledge of appropriate postoperative care, including common analgesics given to rodents and rabbits following surgical

procedures (Champion, Calantropio-Covington, and Sirois, 2022; Suckow, Hashway, Pritchett-Corning, 2023; Suckow and Schroeder, 2010).

- The student displays knowledge of up-to-date guidelines for avoiding, minimizing, and alleviating pain in laboratory animals. The student displays understanding of how to recognize pain and/or distress in rats, mice, and rabbits and demonstrates knowledge of how to implement appropriate pain management protocols, while continuing to monitor the animal's ongoing status. The student demonstrates awareness that any animal given anesthetic and/or analgesic agents must be closely monitored for adverse effects in the pre-anesthetic, anesthetic, and post-procedural periods (AALAS, 2021; Suckow, Hashway, Pritchett-Corning, 2023; Suckow and Schroeder, 2010).

15) **The student accurately identifies and describes common signs of the following diseases in laboratory mice and demonstrates knowledge of which diseases are zoonotic** (AALAS, 2021; Champion, Calantropio-Covington, and Sirois, 2022; Whary et al., 2015; Suckow, Hashway, Pritchett-Corning, 2023):
   a) **Viral**
      - Adenovirus types 1 and 2 (MAV1 and 2)
      - Mouse minute virus (MVM)
      - Epizootic diarrhea of infant mice (EDIM)
   b) **Bacterial**:
      - *Cilia-Associated Respiratory Bacillus* (CAR)
      - *Klebsiella* spp.
      - *Pasturella* spp.
      - *Staphylococcus* spp.
      - *Pseudomonas aeruginosa*
      - *Proteus* spp.
   c) **Parasitic**
      - *Syphacia obvelata* (Pinworm)

- Giardia
- *Myobia musculi* and *Mycoptes musculinus* (mite infestation).

16) **The student accurately identifies and describes common signs of the following diseases in laboratory rats and demonstrates knowledge of which diseases are zoonotic** (AALAS, 2021; Champion, Calantropio-Covington, and Sirois, 2022; Otto, Franklin, and Clifford, 2015):
   a) **Viral:**
      - Adenovirus
      - Mouse minute virus (MVM)
      - Rotavirus
   b) **Bacterial**
      - *Corynebacterium*
      - *Streptococcus* spp.
      - *Pseudomonas aeruginosa*
      - *Staphylococcus* spp.
      - *Proteus* spp.
   c) **Parasitic**
      - *Syphacia muris* (pinworm)
      - *Radforia ensifera* (mite infestation)
      - Entamoeba

17) **The student accurately identifies and describes common signs of the following diseases in laboratory rabbits and demonstrates knowledge of which diseases are zoonotic** (AALAS, 2021; Champion, Calantropio-Covington, and Sirois, 2022; Suckow and Schroeder, 2010):
   a) **Viral**
      - Rotavirus
   b) **Bacterial**
      - *Pasturella multocida*
      - *Clostridium piliforme* (Tyzzer disease)
      - *Clostridium difficile*
   c) **Parasitic**
      - Oxyuriasis (pinworm)
   d) **Mycotic**
      - *Trichophyton mentagrophyte* (ringworm)
   e) **Other**
      - Gastric trichobezoar

References

American Association of Laboratory Animal Science (AALAS). (2021). *Laboratory Animal Technician Training Manual*. Memphis: McNeal Graphics.

Bayne, K. and Anderson, L.C. (2015). Laws, regulations, and policies affecting the use of laboratory animals. In *Laboratory Animal Medicine*, 3rd e. (ed. J. G. Fox, L. C. Anderson, G. Otto, K. R. Pritchett-Corning, and M. T. Whary), 23–42. San Diego: Academic Press.

Champion, J.R., Calantropio-Covington, D., and Sirois, M. (2022). *Laboratory Animal and Exotic Pet Medicine: Principles and Procedures*, 3rd e. (pp. 114–134, 135–152). St. Louis: Elsevier.

National Research Council. (2011). *Guide for the Care and Use of Laboratory Animals*, 8th e. Washington, DC: National Academy Press.

Otto, G. M., Franklin, C. L., and Clifford, C.B. (2015). Biology and diseases of rats. In *Laboratory Animal Medicine*, 3rd e. (ed. J. G. Fox, L. C. Anderson, G. Otto, K. R. Pritchett-Corning, and M. T. Whary), 151–207. San Diego: Academic Press.

Ragland, N. H. (2017). Laboratory animal care and procedures. In *Assessing Essential Skills of Veterinary Technology Students*, 3rd e. (ed. L. J. Buell, L. E. Schenkel, and S. Timperman), 63–67. Ames: John Wiley & Sons, Inc.

Suckow, M. A., Hashway, S. A., and Pritchett-Corning, K. R. (2023). *The Laboratory Mouse*, 3rd e. (pp. 6–7, 55–57, 100–121, 157, 159, 169, 172, 174–188). Boca Raton: CRC Press.

Suckow, M. A., and Schroeder, V. (2010). *The Laboratory Rabbit*, 2nd e. (pp. 9, 25–26, 35–46, 56–60, 63–77, 87–88). Boca Raton: CRC Press.

Whary, M. T., Baumgarth, N., Fox, J. G., and Barthold, S. W. (2015). Biology and diseases of mice. In *Laboratory Animal Medicine,* 3rd e. (ed. J. G. Fox, L. C. Anderson, G. Otto, K. R. Pritchett-Corning, and M. T. Whary), 43–149. San Diego: Academic Press.

9

Avian, Exotic Animal, and Small Mammal Nursing
Annmarie Gonzalez, BS, LVT

1) **The student properly demonstrates an understanding of and performs safe and effective restraint methods for birds.**
   - The student displays knowledge of pertinent avian anatomy and physiology.
   - To help ensure the safety of the patient and handler, the student demonstrates an understanding of the need for specialized restraint techniques for birds.
   - The student displays an appreciation of the importance of minimizing stress in birds and shows knowledge of signs of stress in birds, such as fluffing of feathers, open-beak breathing, and tail bobbing.
   - The student displays the ability to properly restrain birds, grasping around the head, and never grabbing the body or squeezing the chest (pectoral area). The student gently holds the head between the thumb and the forefinger and supports the lower limbs. The student shows awareness that a second handler or tools such as a towel may be needed to restrain the wings and body (Feyrecilde et al., 2021).

2) **The student demonstrates an understanding of and displays the ability to provide client education on particular diets/nutritional concerns for birds, reptiles, amphibians, guinea pigs, hamsters, gerbils, and ferrets.**
   - The student displays knowledge of how the anatomy and physiology of each species determines its nutritional needs.
   - The student displays knowledge that the proper diet for birds depends on species and life stage. The student also shows awareness that feeding an all-seed diet is not recommended for captive birds as it causes deficiencies in vitamin A, calcium, and sodium, and is high in fat. The student demonstrates awareness that fruits can be offered sparingly, because they do not offer protein and may have high sugar and calorie contents. The student displays awareness that commercially available pelleted diets are recommended (Burns, 2021).
   - The student demonstrates awareness that based on order and species, reptiles require widely varying diets, ranging from carnivorous to omnivorous to herbivorous.
   - The student demonstrates awareness that insectivorous reptiles and amphibians eating crickets or mealworms require "gut-loading" diets year-round (a diet of crickets alone is nutritionally inadequate and unacceptable). To determine proper diets for each class, order, and species, the student displays knowledge of appropriate references to consult, such as *Fowler's Zoo and Wild Animal Medicine* (Miller and Fowler, 2015).

Assessing Essential Skills of Veterinary Technology Students, Fourth Edition. Edited by Lisa E. Schenkel, Amanda Colón, Sandra Lynn Bertholf, Sabrina Timperman, and Laurie J. Buell.
© 2024 John Wiley & Sons, Inc. Published 2024 by John Wiley & Sons, Inc.
Companion website: www.wiley.com/go/Schenkel/AssessingEssentialSkillsofVeterinaryTechnologyStudents4e

- Regarding guinea pigs, the student demonstrates knowledge that the recommended diet for pet guinea pigs meets requirements for the high fiber and moderate protein levels provided by commercial guinea pig pellets and a free choice of high-quality timothy grass hay (Pignon and Mayer, 2021).
- The student displays awareness that guinea pigs need daily vitamin C supplementation (approximate daily requirements for adults are 10–25 mg/kg daily for maintenance and 30 mg/kg daily for growing and pregnant guinea pigs) (Pignon and Mayer, 2021).
- The student demonstrates an understanding that over-the-counter vitamin C water additives should not be used as they can alter the taste of the water, dissuading the animal from consuming enough water.
- The student also displays awareness that fresh foods containing vitamin C should be offered in small amounts. However, vegetables containing oxalates, such as kale, parsley, and beet greens, should not be offered, since they can contribute to the formation of urinary calculi (Burns, 2021).
- The student displays awareness that the vitamin C contained in commercial pellets expires 90 days after the date of manufacture (Pignon and Mayer, 2021).
- Regarding hamsters, the student demonstrates knowledge that nutritionally balanced pelleted diets specifically formulated for hamsters with 14% to 17% protein are recommended with small amounts of fresh leafy greens. The student also displays awareness that seed-mixed-with-pellet diets are not recommended as the main diet since they can lead to selective eating and thus, nutritional deficiencies and obesity. The student demonstrates awareness that hamsters in the wild are omnivorous (Burns, 2021).
- Regarding gerbils, the student displays awareness that commercial gerbil pellets with up to 22% protein, along with a small amount of fresh leafy greens, are recommended, but seed mixes are not nutritionally adequate and therefore, not recommended. The student also demonstrates awareness that gerbils develop high cholesterol levels when placed on a high-fat, high-cholesterol diet (Miwa and Mayer, 2021).
- Regarding ferrets, the student displays the recognition that they are strict carnivores and that complete diet requirements are unknown. The student shows awareness that commercially available ferret diets or cat diets containing quality and highly digestible protein and fat and low in complex carbohydrates (including sugar and fiber) are acceptable diets for ferrets (Kollias and Fernandez-Moran 2015).
- The student shows knowledge of the consequences of feeding each species an inappropriate and/or inadequate diet.
- The student displays knowledge of how to safely obtain subjective and objective data to recognize abnormal behavior patterns that may arise from inadequate nutrition.
- The student explains the nutritional needs and the importance of proper diets for birds, reptiles, amphibians, guinea pigs, hamsters, gerbils, and ferrets clearly and succinctly and in a manner understandable to the client.
- The student recommends appropriate references such as texts, educational websites, and clinical education materials to the client.

3) **The student demonstrates an understanding of and displays the ability to provide client education regarding the particular water needs of birds, reptiles, amphibians, guinea pigs, hamsters, gerbils, and ferrets.**
   - The student displays knowledge of how the physiology of each species determines its water needs and how each species obtains water in its natural and captive environment.
   - The student demonstrates awareness, depending on the species, that adequate

fresh water, cleaned daily or more frequently, should be available at all times.

- The student displays knowledge that some birds, in addition to drinking water, require a bird bath that should be emptied, cleaned, and refreshed daily.
- The student demonstrates awareness that amphibians and some reptiles also require bathing/basking pools that should be emptied, cleaned, and refreshed daily.
- The student displays knowledge that, for guinea pigs, hamsters, gerbils, and ferrets, adequate amounts of fresh water should be available in sipper bottles that are checked for proper function and cleaned daily.
- The student displays knowledge of how to safely obtain subjective and objective data to recognize abnormal behavior patterns that may arise from inadequate hydration.
- The student explains water needs for birds, reptiles, amphibians, guinea pigs, hamsters, gerbils, and ferrets clearly and succinctly, and in a manner understandable to the client.
- The student recommends appropriate references such as texts, educational websites, and clinical education materials to the client.

4) **The student demonstrates an understanding of and displays the ability to provide client education regarding the particular caging/aquarium needs of birds, reptiles, amphibians, guinea pigs, hamsters, gerbils, and ferrets.**
    - The student shows familiarity with the importance of (1) exposing the bird to fresh air and unfiltered sunlight (and/or a full spectrum UV light source) at least 20 minutes twice weekly; (2) misting the bird frequently to encourage grooming and hydration; and (3) providing the opportunity for a water bath or shower.
    - The student displays an understanding of how to choose an appropriate location for the cage/aquarium to provide a safe and comfortable environment for the animal.
    - The student shows an understanding that birds require cages that are as large as

possible; at minimum, the cage should be large enough to allow the bird to spread its wings without touching the sides. The student demonstrates awareness that the cage should be frequently cleaned (to remove organic debris) and disinfected with a 1:10 diluted solution of white vinegar and water (Heatley and Cornejo, 2015). The student displays awareness that many other household cleansers should not be used because they may emit fumes that are toxic to birds.

- The student displays familiarity with appropriate cage substrates and perches of varying diameter (i.e., to help prevent chronic inflammatory conditions of the foot or bumblefoot), and the need to replace substrates and perches frequently (i.e., when soiled).
- The student demonstrates awareness that, since natural habitats of reptiles and amphibians vary widely, housing should mirror the natural environment as closely as possible (including light, temperature, humidity, ventilation, etc.). The student displays knowledge of appropriate references to consult for the proper environment, caging/aquarium, and caging substrate for each class, order, and species.
- The student displays awareness of the contraindications of certain substrates for reptiles. For example, sand can cause an impaction in certain species due to ingestion of the sand.
- The student demonstrates an understanding of the importance of exposing reptiles to full spectrum UV light for the appropriate time period depending on species.
- The student shows knowledge that exposure of reptiles to direct sunlight is ideal. The student displays cognizance that exposure to sunlight through glass is inadequate and that, if a reptile is placed in a glass enclosure outdoors, death may result from rapidly elevating lethal temperatures. The student also displays awareness that the UVB output of full-spectrum UV lamps needs to be

measured periodically in order to determine if the lamp no longer emits adequate UVB light and needs to be replaced (Baines and Cusack, 2019).

- The student displays knowledge that some amphibians are highly susceptible to water toxins and pH changes (due to skin permeability), necessitating daily skin inspections. The student also shows awareness that some lungless amphibians depend on cutaneous respiration (Baitchman and Herman, 2015).
- For ferrets, guinea pigs, hamsters, and gerbils, the student displays knowledge of appropriate caging, cage substrates, lighting, ventilation, cage size, and the need to provide accessories and/or materials for nesting, climbing, exercising, and/or hiding.
- For ferrets, guinea pigs, hamsters, and gerbils, the student displays awareness of the importance of daily cleaning of the cage and cage substrate.
- The student demonstrates awareness that cages or pens for ferrets must be large enough for exercise and, to reduce stress, cages should include dark areas for sleeping, such as suitable, commercially available cloth hammocks and cage shelves. Cardboard or plastic can be used if a ferret is known to eat fabric. In addition, when outside of their cages or pens, ferrets should not be left unsupervised and, due to their propensity to chew almost anything, the home should be "ferret-proofed." The student displays awareness that ferrets may be trained to use litter boxes. Pelleted litter rather than clay or clumping litter is recommended (Powers and Perpiñán, 2021).
- The student displays knowledge that aquaria or metal cages with solid floors are suitable for guinea pigs because of their very soft feet, which are prone to injury if housed in cages with wire bottoms. The student shows knowledge that appropriate cage substrates include newspaper or shredded paper. In addition, the student displays awareness that for hamsters and gerbils, hardwood chips or recycled paper pellets are suitable cage substrates, but synthetic, commercial nesting materials are not recommended because they may injure the feet or cause impaction if ingested.

- The student displays awareness that guinea pigs enjoy being housed with other guinea pigs, but hamsters and gerbils are best housed singly.
- For birds, reptiles, amphibians, guinea pigs, hamsters, gerbils, and ferrets, the student displays knowledge of how to safely obtain subjective and objective data to recognize abnormal behavior patterns that may arise from inappropriate caging and substrate.
- The student explains caging/aquarium needs for birds, reptiles, amphibians, guinea pigs, hamsters, gerbils, and ferrets clearly and succinctly in a manner understandable to the client.
- The student recommends appropriate references such as texts, educational websites, and clinical education materials to the client.

5) **The student demonstrates an understanding of and displays the ability to provide client education regarding the reproduction of birds, reptiles, amphibians, guinea pigs, hamsters, gerbils, and ferrets.**

- In general, the student demonstrates familiarity with species-specific breeding requirements, including environmental and dietary adjustments necessitated by pregnancy and/or lactation.
- The student displays knowledge of the anatomy and physiology of reproduction in the various species.
- The student demonstrates awareness of how to sex various species (when possible) and their specific breeding requirements.
- The student displays knowledge of common causes and clinical signs of dystocia in the various species, such as improper nutrition. For example, a cockatiel on an

all-seed diet is at high risk of becoming egg-bound due to hypocalcemia.

- The student shows awareness of the complications of dystocia and the need for immediate veterinary attention.
- The student displays knowledge that some birds have difficulty laying eggs and many of these are first-time egg layers. In addition, the student shows awareness that certain species are more prone to becoming chronic egg layers, leading to an increased risk for hypocalcemia and egg binding.
- The student displays knowledge that the presence of a male is not necessary to stimulate egg-laying behavior in a female bird.
- The student shows awareness that the presence of a male is not necessary for egg production in some species of reptiles and amphibians.
- The student demonstrates awareness that reptiles can be egg-laying or viviparous. The student shows familiarity with the proper temperature and humidity for egg incubation and clinical signs of "egg-bound" females.
- The student displays awareness that amphibians can be oviparous, viviparous, and ovoviviparous (Klaphake, 2010).
- The student demonstrates knowledge that guinea pigs breed best in monogamous pairs, but pregnant sows must be separated from other adults until the litter is weaned. The student shows awareness that guinea pigs are prone to dystocia due to narrow pelvic canals and pups that tend to be large in size. Sows bred after seven to eight months of age have a higher incidence of dystocia (Pignon and Mayer, 2021).
- The student shows knowledge that hamsters should be bred by placing the female in the male's cage one hour before dark and removing her after mating or when fighting ensues. The student displays awareness that cannibalism of the young is common in hamsters; however, fostering and hand-raising of the young is not recommended.
- The student shows awareness that gerbils are non-seasonally polyestrous and prefer monogamous pairing, with the male helping to raise the young (Champion, Calantropio-Covington, and Sirois, 2022).
- The student displays knowledge that intact female ferrets, or jills, are induced ovulators with a 41- to 42-day gestation period. The student shows an understanding that females who are not intended to be bred should be spayed because, if not bred, females usually remain in heat, which can cause fatal, estrogen-induced anemia (Champion, Calantropio-Covington, and Sirois, 2022).
- The student explains pertinent reproduction for birds, reptiles, amphibians, guinea pigs, hamsters, gerbils, and ferrets clearly and succinctly in a manner understandable to the client.
- The student recommends appropriate references such as texts, educational websites, and clinical education materials to the client.

6) **The student demonstrates an understanding of and displays the ability to provide client education on the particular grooming needs of birds, reptiles, amphibians, guinea pigs, hamsters, gerbils, and ferrets.**

- The student demonstrates knowledge of proper techniques for beak, wing, and nail clipping. The student shows awareness that the goal of wing clipping is prevention of sustained flight as opposed to making the bird unable to fly (Arent and Franzen-Klein, 2024).
- The student demonstrates knowledge that reptiles vary greatly in grooming requirements. In addition, the student demonstrates an understanding that the handling of reptiles should be avoided during shedding (ecdysis), and excessively low humidity is associated with dysecdysis (Champion, Calantropio-Covington, and Sirois, 2022).
- The student demonstrates knowledge of the appropriate way shedding (ecdysis)

normally occurs in various reptiles. For example, snakes shed their skins in one piece whereas certain species of lizards can shed their skins in multiple pieces.

- The student shows awareness that the clouding of eyes in reptiles is an indication of impending shedding.
- The student demonstrates knowledge that small mammals have varying needs for basic grooming. For example, ferrets may require ear-cleaning, toenail trimming, and dental prophylaxis. As another example, because the incisors and molars of guinea pigs grow continuously, the teeth may require trimming.
- The student shows awareness that guinea pigs may need toenail trimming, and long-haired breeds need brushing.
- For birds, reptiles, amphibians, guinea pigs, hamsters, gerbils, and ferrets, the student displays knowledge of how to safely obtain subjective and objective data to recognize abnormal behavior patterns that may arise from inappropriate grooming.
- The student explains basic grooming for birds, reptiles, amphibians, guinea pigs, hamsters, gerbils, and ferrets clearly and succinctly in a manner understandable to the client.
- The student recommends appropriate references such as texts, educational websites, and clinical education materials to the client.

7) **The student demonstrates an understanding of and displays the ability to provide client education regarding the proper transportation methods for birds, reptiles, amphibians, guinea pigs, hamsters, gerbils, and ferrets.**
   - The student displays the ability to describe appropriate transportation methods for various species, based on the knowledge that the stress of inappropriate travel methods can seriously affect patient health.
   - The student displays knowledge of appropriate methods for transporting birds, with the awareness that they should be

protected from excessive heat or cold and not left unattended in cars.
- The student demonstrates awareness that reptiles and amphibians should be transported either in their own caging/aquaria or in a similar, but more compact, enclosure that contains some substrate and is kept covered and warm, protected from temperature extremes, and not left unattended in a car. In addition, the student displays knowledge that amphibians should be lightly misted with warm water prior to transport.
- The student shows knowledge that rodents may be transported in their own cages (or smaller cages if their usual habitats are too large), and a sheet or towel may be used to cover the cage to reduce visual stressors. The student demonstrates knowledge that the cage should be protected from excessive heat or cold and not left in an unattended car.
- The student demonstrates awareness that ferrets may be transported safely in cat carriers.
- The student explains appropriate transportation methods for birds, reptiles, amphibians, guinea pigs, hamsters, gerbils, and ferrets clearly and succinctly in a manner understandable to the client.
- The student recommends appropriate references such as texts, educational websites, and clinical education materials to the client.

8) **The student demonstrates knowledge of and displays the ability to provide client education regarding the clinical role of proper husbandry in maintaining the well-being of birds, reptiles, amphibians, guinea pigs, hamsters, gerbils, and ferrets.**
   - The student shows awareness that the majority of disease states in these species are due to improper husbandry.
   - The student recognizes inappropriate husbandry of the various species such as improper nutrition and environment.
   - The student displays knowledge of normal behavior patterns of the various

species. The student displays the ability to recognize abnormal behavior patterns.

- For birds, reptiles, amphibians, guinea pigs, hamsters, gerbils, and ferrets, the student displays knowledge of how to safely obtain subjective and objective data to recognize abnormal behavior patterns that may arise from inappropriate husbandry.
- The student explains the clinical role of proper husbandry for birds, reptiles, amphibians, guinea pigs, hamsters, gerbils, and ferrets clearly and succinctly in a manner understandable to the client.
- The student recommends appropriate references such as texts, educational websites, and clinical education materials to the client.

9) **The student collects objective data on birds in the form of an avian exam.**
- Prior to beginning the physical exam, the student observes the bird's behavior and appearance in the cage. In addition, the student accurately determines the respiratory rate and character while the bird is at rest.
- The student chooses the appropriate method for weighing the bird based on the bird's behavior and condition and obtains an accurate weight.
- The student uses appropriate restraint techniques.
- The student correctly examines the head, displaying awareness that the top of the head should be smooth (matted feathers may be a sign of illness), eyes should be clear and open, and touching the medial canthus should cause a blink reflex. The student checks the eyes for symmetry, discharge, or redness and gently lifts the eyelid to subjectively monitor for hydration as the lid resumes its normal location.
- The student properly examines the cere and nostrils, displaying knowledge that the cere should be smooth and soft, the nostrils should be clear, free of discharge, and symmetrical, and the operculum within the nares should be free

of abnormal accumulation. The student correctly locates and examines the ears by gently parting the feathers on each side of the head. The student shows awareness that the beak should be smooth, shiny, and of normal length. The student then properly inserts an oral speculum to examine the oral cavity, assessing the choanal slit and its papillae, as well as the color and moistness of the oral mucosa. The student palpates the crop for abnormalities.
- The student observes and accurately determines the respiratory rate during restraint, showing understanding that, after examination, a healthy bird should resume its pre-handling respiratory rate within minutes. The student displays awareness that respiratory rates and heart rates are faster in smaller birds than larger birds. Using a pediatric stethoscope, the student auscultates the heart, accurately determining the heart rate.
- The student displays an understanding of and the ability to correctly determine the "body condition score." The student properly palpates the pectoral muscles and abdomen.
- The student properly extends the wings and carefully palpates the bones, joints, and patagium.
- The student properly examines the cloaca and everts it, if possible, to examine the cloacal mucosa. The student correctly examines the uropygial gland in birds that have one.
- The student properly examines the feathers over the entire body, as well as the skin of the feet, and also checks the nails for overgrowth.

10) **The student participates in the procedure of correctly performing an avian nail trim.**
- The student displays knowledge of the nail anatomy of common avian species.
- The student correctly restrains the bird for the nail trim.

- The student explains appropriate equipment and technique for an avian nail trim.
- The student demonstrates the ability to properly hold both guillotine and scissors-type nail clippers, Dremel Motor Tools, or files; estimates the location of the vascular matrix; correctly trims nails; and applies cauterization agents/hemostatic techniques when needed.

References

Arent, L. R., and Franzen-Klein, D. (2024). Avian anatomy and physiology. In *Clinical Anatomy and Physiology for Veterinary Technicians*, 4th e. (ed. T. Colville and J. M. Bassert), 547. St. Louis: Elsevier.

Baines, F. M., and Cusack, L. M. (2019). Environmental lighting. In *Mader's Reptile and Amphibian Medicine and Surgery* (ed. S. J. Stahl and S. J. Divers), 131. St. Louis: Elsevier.

Baitchman E. J. and Herman T.A. (2015). Caudata (Urodela): Tailed amphibians. In *Fowler's Zoo and Wild Animal Medicine*, 8th e. (ed. R. E. Miller and M. E. Fowler), 14. St. Louis: Elsevier.

Burns, K. M. (2021). Animal nutrition. In *McCurnin's Clinical Textbook for Veterinary Technicians and Nurses*, 10th e. (ed. J. M. Bassert, A. D. Beal, O. M. Samples), 313–318. St. Louis: Elsevier.

Champion, J.R., Calantropio-Covington, D. and Sirois, M. (2022). Reptiles. In *Laboratory Animal and Exotic Pet Medicine*, 3rd e. (ed. M. Sirois), 82–99. St. Louis: Elsevier.

Heatley, J. J. and Cornejo, J. (2015). Psittaciformes. In *Fowler's Zoo and Wild Animal Medicine*, 8th e. (ed. R. E. Miller and M. E. Fowler), 172. St. Louis: Elsevier.

Feyrecilde, M., Guiberson, J., and Temple Grandin (2021). Restraint and Handling of Animals. In *McCurnin's Clinical Textbook for Veterinary Technicians and Nurses*, 10th e. (ed. J. M. Bassert, A. D. Beal, O. M. Samples, 204–206. St. Louis: Elsevier.

Klaphake, E. (2010). Reproductive disease in reptiles and amphibians. *American Board of Veterinary Practitioners Symposium 2010 Proceedings Online*. Denver: American Board of Veterinary Practitioners.

Kollias, G. V. and Fernandez-Moran, J. (2015). Mustelidae. In *Fowler's Zoo and Wild Animal Medicine*, 8th e. (ed. R. E. Miller and M. E. Fowler), 172. 480. St. Louis: Elsevier.

Miller, R. E., & Fowler, M. E. (2015). *Fowler's Zoo and Wild Animal Medicine*, 8th e. St. Louis: Elsevier.

Miwa, Y. and Mayer, J. (2021). Hamster and gerbils. In *Ferrets, Rabbits, and Rodents Clinical Medicine and Surgery* (ed. K. E. Quesenberry, C. J. Orcutt, C. Mans, and J. W. Carpenter), 371. St. Louis: Elsevier.

Pignon, C. and Mayer, J. (2021). Guinea pig. In *Ferrets, Rabbits, and Rodents Clinical Medicine and Surgery* (ed. K. E. Quesenberry, C. J. Orcutt, C. Mans, and J. W. Carpenter), 274. St. Louis: Elsevier.

Powers, L. V. and Perpiñán, D. (2021). Basic anatomy, physiology, and husbandry of ferrets. In *Ferrets, Rabbits, and Rodents Clinical Medicine and Surgery* (ed. K. E. Quesenberry, C. J. Orcutt, C. Mans, and J. W. Carpenter), 10. St. Louis: Elsevier.

Timperman, S., Schenkel, L. E., Buell, L. J., and Gamez C. J. (2017). Avian and exotic animal nursing. In *Assessing Essential Skills of Veterinary Technology Students*, 3rd e. (ed. L. J. Buell, L. E. Schenkel, and S. Timperman), 69–74. Ames: John Wiley & Sons, Inc.

Index

Assessing Essential Skills of Veterinary Technology Students, Fourth Edition. Edited by Lisa E. Schenkel,
Amanda Colón, Sandra Lynn Bertholf, Sabrina Timperman, and Laurie J. Buell.
© 2024 John Wiley & Sons, Inc. Published 2024 by John Wiley & Sons, Inc.
Companion website: www.wiley.com/go/Schenkel/AssessingEssentialSkillsofVeterinaryTechnologyStudents4e